Getting into University

Physiotherapy Courses

Aaron Ghuman

12th edition

trotman | **t**

Getting into University: Physiotherapy Courses

This 12th edition published in 2025 by Trotman, an imprint of Trotman Indigo Publishing Ltd, 18e Charles Street, Bath BA1 1HX

© Trotman Indigo Publishing Ltd 2025

Author: Aaron Ghuman
11th edn: James Griffith
10th–9th edns: Philip Shanahan
8th–5th edns: James Barton
4th edn: James Burnett
3rd edn: James Burnett & Maya Waterstone
2nd–1st edns: James Burnett & Andrew Long

British Library Cataloguing in Publication Data
A catalogue record for this book is available from the British Library.

Paperback ISBN 978 1 911724 46 9
eISBN 978 1 911724 47 6

Every effort has been made to trace copyright holders and to obtain their permission for the use of copyright material. The publisher apologises for any errors or omissions, and would be grateful to be notified of any corrections that should be incorporated in future editions of this book.

The authorised representative in the EEA is Easy Access System Europe Oü (EAS), Mustamäe tee 50, 10621 Tallinn, Estonia.

Printed and bound in the UK by 4Edge Ltd, Hockley, Essex

All details in this book were correct at the time of going to press. To keep up to date with all the latest news and updates and to access the online resources that accompany this book, use this QR code or visit www.trotman.co.uk/pages/getting-into-online-resources.

Contents

About the author

Aaron Ghuman is a Director of Recruitment for the Mander Portman Woodward (MPW) in Birmingham. As a member of the Senior Leadership Team, Aaron interviews students as part of their admissions process to MPW, offering advice on the right study path to take for their dream university and course.

Acknowledgements

Many thanks are due to all those who have written previous editions of *Getting into University: Physiotherapy Courses*.

I would also like to especially thank the Chartered Society of Physiotherapy (CSP) for the huge amount of information they provided for the completion of this book.

The information in this book has come from a variety of sources and is, I believe, correct at the time of going to press. However, the views expressed are my own and any errors are down to me.

I hope that you find this book a valuable and helpful source, and I wish you all the success in your future endeavours in physiotherapy.

Aaron Ghuman
January 2025

Warming up

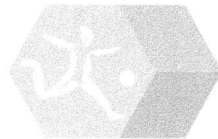

Introduction

Football 2022. Chloe Kelly's promising football career faced a significant setback during a Women's Super League match between Manchester City and Birmingham City. While pressing in the attacking third, Kelly awkwardly twisted her knee after an aggressive challenge. She collapsed in visible pain, clutching her leg, and had to be stretchered off the pitch. Chloe suffered an anterior cruciate ligament (ACL) rupture, one of the most severe injuries in sport, with a recovery timeline often stretching to a year or more. For any athlete, this could have been a career-defining blow.

However, what followed was a story of resilience and determination. With the unwavering support of her physiotherapy team, Kelly embarked on an intense and structured rehabilitation programme. The process included strength-building exercises, proprioception drills to restore balance and coordination, and carefully monitored reintroduction to the high-intensity demands of elite football.

Fast forward to the summer of 2022, Kelly spectacularly returned to the spotlight. During the UEFA Women's European Championship final, she scored the winning goal in extra time, sealing England's historic victory over Germany. Her joyful celebration became the iconic image of the tournament.

Athletics 2024. The 2024 Summer Olympics in Paris highlighted the vital contributions of physiotherapists in ensuring athletes could perform at their best. Team GB's medical support team, which included multiple physiotherapists and doctors, played a key role in delivering tailored care to the athletes.

Most people associate physiotherapy with sport and the injuries of high-profile sportsmen and women. For instance, it is not uncommon on a Monday morning, when flicking through the back pages of the paper, to see that the physiotherapist is assessing Johnny X after having sustained a knock in the weekend's Premiership match. It is a physiotherapist's job to rehabilitate the multi-million-pound stars from their bumps and cuts (and broken bones, torn ligaments, muscle damage etc.).

At the other end of the scale, physiotherapy can be used to correct smaller injuries, for example, those sustained in an accident when the victim needs to learn to walk properly again. It has also gained prominence as a profession because of the leading role it has taken in the armed forces and the rehabilitation work it does with soldiers who have been injured in the line of duty, allowing them to lead normal lives after what are life-altering injuries, and this work needs to be reflected.

In short, physios are invaluable.

Never before has physiotherapy been so much in the media attention; whether from initiatives to get the UK moving and deal with growing health issues or with physiotherapists having an increased role in the management of a sports team with power of veto and sports stars being suspended for arguing with their decisions. There are also the difficulties the profession faces, with issues ranging from an ageing population to the rise in obesity, to cuts in services. There are many other facets to the profession outside of the treatment room, and admissions tutors require you to be fully aware of that.

I regularly counsel students on their A level subject choices in line with their talents and their desired onward university degree. Few are aware of how competitive physiotherapy is, particularly, as they may be weighing this degree choice up against something else like medicine. I hope this book will provide a better understanding on the benefits of studying physiotherapy at undergraduate level and how to make a competitive application in order to obtain a place.

Physiotherapy is a popular degree, and some universities have cut the number of places on offer, meaning that there is now even greater competition for places. Table 1 shows you the proportion of applications that received an offer to study physiotherapy.

What is physiotherapy?

The human body is a complex machine that can go wrong for any number of reasons. Physiotherapy is a science-based medical subject that looks in detail at how the body moves; how muscles, bones, joints and ligaments work; and how they react to pain and

Table 1: Proportion of applications that received an offer to study physiotherapy

Year	Proportion of applications receiving offer
2019	34.7%
2020	36.2%
2021	31.6%
2022	26.6%
2023	29.5%

Source: UCAS undergraduate end-of-year cycle data 2023.

trauma. Physiotherapists diagnose numerous ailments that affect the muscles and nerves and then proceed to treat the patient, ensuring independence, movement and a return to maximum performance. It is the physiotherapist's job not only to look at the problem and treat it but also to look for any predisposing factors that may have contributed to the patient's ailment and to advise on how to minimise the risk of the same thing happening again.

Qualified physiotherapists work both independently and as part of multidisciplinary teams, ensuring that patients' health and mobility are improved.

What do physiotherapists do?

Physiotherapists have numerous challenging roles within the health sector. They provide services such as rehabilitation and exercise before and after surgery. Within the wider community, they provide services to adults with learning difficulties. They also have a role in the workplace where they can help to reduce injuries such as repetitive strain injury (RSI).

Chartered physiotherapists work with a wide range of people in many different environments, either individually or as part of a large healthcare team;

Physiotherapists deal with many different situations, including the following:

- educating patients is very important in physiotherapy and means teaching people the 'correct' way to move and lift in order to prevent or slow the onset of problems such as back pain or RSI (see Chapter 7). This may include helping athletes to avoid injury by discussing techniques and training programmes. Poor warm-up routines, too much training, poor equipment and incorrect technique are common causes of injuries, and all of these can be avoided. Using the idea that prevention is better than cure, physiotherapists are able to show people that very small changes will be hugely beneficial, for example, good footwear or the use of wrist support when using a computer.
- helping women before and after pregnancy by advising them about posture and exercise;
- helping children to deal with mental and physical disabilities;
- developing the potential of people with learning difficulties through exercise, sport and recreation; this could also include the use of specialist equipment;
- helping stroke victims to recover movement in paralysed limbs;
- helping heart attack victims to reduce the risk of future recurrence;

- helping orthopaedic patients after spinal operations or joint replacements and treating those debilitated following an accident. Using a variety of techniques to strengthen muscles and improve the mobility of individual joints, activities such as walking can be made much easier for people recovering from hip replacements or those with arthritis or osteoporosis. These methods can also reduce the pain and stiffness resulting from these conditions.
- working with AIDS patients;
- caring for those people who suffer from Parkinson's disease (one in 37 people in the UK will be diagnosed with Parkinson's disease at some point in their life);
- helping people to deal with stress and anxiety;
- improving the confidence and self-esteem of those with mental illness through exercise and recreation, while also helping with relaxation and body-awareness techniques;
- working with the terminally ill (both inpatients and outpatients) or those in intensive care to maintain movement and prevent respiratory problems;
- helping sportspeople recover from injury;
- working in large businesses and companies to ensure that employees do not suffer from physical problems associated with their jobs.

Physiotherapists use a range of techniques, including:

- exercise;
- hydrotherapy (see Glossary);
- infrared and ultraviolet radiation (see Glossary);
- manipulation;
- massage;
- ultrasound (see Glossary);
- vibration;
- patient education;
- movement analysis;
- gait re-education (see Glossary);
- heat and cold application.

About this book

This book is structured very much like a standard physiotherapy session: it requires adequate warm-up, intensive drills and jumping through hoops before finally seeing the finishing line, only for you to be given a leaflet detailing specific exercises for you to do at home. Stretch and challenge your mind, without breaking your back!

How to use this book

The competition for places on approved degree courses is intense – there are very few university courses other than physiotherapy that have more applicants per place. For example, the University of Birmingham, which ranks first in the Complete University Guide rankings (2025), only offered a place for one in five students who applied to this course. With such intense competition for places, you need to think carefully about all the stages of your application: from the preparation that you do before you apply through to the interview. You should also think about the steps you can take to maximise your chances of gaining a place should something go wrong at the examination stage.

This book covers the following:

- what physiotherapists do;
- getting an interview;
- getting an offer;
- results day;
- useful information.

The book begins with outlining what physiotherapists do and looks at the kind of career you can expect as a physiotherapist. It also describes what the study of physiotherapy involves and the different course structures on offer. Please note that this book is designed to be a route map for potential physiotherapists rather than a comprehensive guide to physiotherapy as a profession. The CSP, or physiotherapists you meet during work experience, should be the starting points for more detailed information on what being a physiotherapist entails.

The book then goes on to deal with the preparation that you need to undertake in order to make your application as strong as possible. It includes advice on work experience, how to choose a university and the UCAS application itself. Information for students with Scottish Highers, the International Baccalaureate (IB), the BTEC National Diploma or the Irish Leaving Certificate is on page 35.

It then covers interviews and provides tips on what to expect and on how to ensure that you come across as a potential physiotherapist. The book also contains a checklist for you to tick off the important steps in making your application.

The 'Results day' chapter describes the steps that you need to take if you are holding an offer or if you do not have an offer but want to gain a place through Clearing. In Chapter 9, there is advice and information for 'non-standard' applicants – mature students, graduates and retake students.

Further to this, the book provides useful information on fees and funding and details of the universities offering courses, including their entry requirements. The universities will be happy to provide you with further information on other qualifications.

To conclude, there is a further information section and a glossary. Here you will find details of sources of further information on physiotherapy and definitions of any terms and abbreviations relevant to your UCAS application for Physiotherapy courses.

1 | Pressure points
Careers

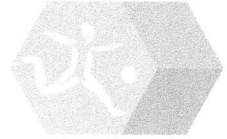

The book's aim is to make sure that you are completely well versed with the fundamentals of physiotherapy before you apply for university study; that includes knowing about the different career opportunities available to you in this profession. The field you are hoping to enter offers a great deal of options and exciting pathways.

It is equally important, when you have qualified for the profession, that you are quite open-minded in your approach and progressive in terms of your thinking. Physiotherapists normally work autonomously, as they are able to accept referrals from a range of sources (though professional autonomy is only granted to CSP members), and therefore you have to consider the business elements of the profession, that is, balancing treatment with an understanding of how to balance the books. What this means is that physiotherapists make their own clinical judgements and treatment decisions, and they also work in reflection, that is, reviewing themselves and making corrections to their work where necessary.

Physiotherapy is a career that relies on the strength of the individual as well as the ability to work in a team. Physiotherapy as a subject is highly academic and therefore of great value; this means that employment prospects are large and varied. These prospects are not limited to the NHS; there is an enormous breadth of employment prospects that can be found across the different sectors (see pages 9–11).

Physiotherapy is not, however, a profession that involves only physical therapy. Physiotherapists work with people – in most cases, people who are disabled or who have been ill or injured. Physiotherapists need to be able to communicate on a personal level with people of all ages, to be reassuring and comforting, to explain the treatments they are using and to help patients overcome fear and pain. Physiotherapists need to be able to assess the needs of their patients and to be aware of the effects of external circumstances such as social or cultural factors.

Working as a physiotherapist

Physiotherapists work in a wide range of health and care environments that include hospitals, the local community, private practice, industry and sports settings. The NHS is the largest employer of physiotherapists in the UK. Physiotherapy comprises the largest group within the allied healthcare professions, with approximately 56,300 (2024) state-registered physiotherapists in the UK, which compares to 44,000 in 2010.

A typical working day depends on whether you are working in the NHS or private practice. In the majority of cases, physiotherapists work in hospitals with normal working days, that is, 9am–5pm, Monday–Friday. There are occasions when a weekend may be required, but this is symptomatic of the health professions.

The most identifiable example is of a hospital physiotherapist working in the physiotherapy department. A calendar booking system is in operation, as in a GP surgery, where they will see many patients per day, each one for an allotted period of time, about a range of problems, such as rehabilitation from broken bones, bad backs and arthritis, for a range of ages.

Those working in hospitals might work on the wards and visit the ward staff to discuss the treatment plans of new patients. Sometimes they then treat them as part of their ongoing care, often taking them to the physiotherapy department. A ward physiotherapist might have half a dozen wards to cover, varying from children's wards to orthopaedic wards or stroke units. In some cases, a physiotherapist might be required to work in the intensive care unit if it is thought essential to the immediate rehabilitation of a patient.

Physiotherapists in private practice may have more opportunities to travel, depending on the job they are doing. If you work for a professional sporting association, for example, you may find that you have to travel a lot to support the team. Sometimes patients will be referred to you; other times you will need to target your business, and that may require advertising.

The concept of travel is also becoming more common in the NHS as a result of changes, as physiotherapists are doing more home visits to support the elderly.

To qualify as a registered physiotherapist, you need to gain an approved degree (see page 17) that has been validated by the CSP and the Health and Care Professions Council (HCPC). If you complete the degree, you must then register with the HCPC to use the professional title of physiotherapist, and you are eligible for membership of the CSP.

As with any career, there are pros and cons to physiotherapy. It is up to you to decide if the pros outweigh the cons. That is why work experience is invaluable, as it will either confirm your decision to pursue the career or demonstrate to you that you should seek an alternative occupation. Physiotherapists have a lot of demands on their time, and they often can be stretched to the limit – if you will excuse the pun – because of the nature of their work, especially within the NHS, where, as a result of staffing cuts, there is more work for an individual physiotherapist. However, the variety and nature of the work is what physiotherapists thrive on, and it is a hugely rewarding career, as you get to see the continuing progress of an individual patient over time.

The question of what attributes a physiotherapist needs is a common one. It is easy to say 'be physically fit'; at the end of the day, practise what you teach. Not to be flippant, it is a good point, as in any very demanding job that requires you to be on your feet most of the day, you want to make sure that you are looking after yourself. Additionally, you also need to consider the psychology of the patient. As with the relationship between a client and a personal trainer in a gym, a patient will have more confidence in their instructor if they can see that the instructor takes good care of themselves. Being active is also necessary for clear thinking, as it gives you the energy to get through the week.

However, over and above that, there are other characteristics that define a good physiotherapist. You need to have patience, peace of mind, the strength of character to encourage a patient and firmness to make sure that they achieve their targets. A physiotherapist is a strategist. Each individual will find their own style – and you should be encouraged to find yours – but it all comes from this foundation, and you need to consider now whether you possess those attributes.

Common career paths for physiotherapists

Once you have completed your BSc in Physiotherapy, you will, hopefully, gain membership of the CSP and become registered with the HCPC – all degree courses in the UK are now accredited by the CSP and the HCPC. To say that there is a standard route is not correct. The main thing you need after graduating is clinical experience, and the usual route will be to gain experience in areas that you did not cover on your placements, usually as a junior in a rotational band 5 job with a starting salary of £29,969.

A rotational band 5 job is a general physiotherapist role in which you rotate through the various departments in a hospital, including respiratory, stroke, orthopaedic and so on. Each rotation will last around four months. These are commonly in the NHS or in some private practices and are designed to build up your expertise before you can qualify for the next band (band 6). These bands also equate to your pay scale.

A lot of physiotherapists get their rotational band 5 job through the NHS or by having impressed on their placements during their course. However, you do not have to have worked for the NHS first before going into private practice. Some physiotherapists set up their own practices, but their success is all based on reputation and on building up the relevant experience over many years. As for anything in life, you have to prove yourself first.

Further qualifications are not essential after your degree, but you are expected to maintain your continuing professional development (CPD), which is very important and discussed below.

Private practice is one of the more lucrative career moves. Private practice, as an umbrella term, includes:

- treating patients independently for the same ailments as in the NHS;
- working for a sports club or a specific team, aiding in the recovery of sportspersons from injury and helping to optimise their performance;
- occupational rehabilitation, which means helping people to recover from accidents or illnesses and to return to their normal lives.

There are also additional opportunities to go off on a tangent and get involved in policy development and research in order to ensure that physiotherapy as a profession continues to progress over time in line with NHS changes and guidelines.

Some of the other areas of work available to you as an aspiring physiotherapist are outlined in Table 2.

Employment prospects

In 2023, the CSP reported: 'In the UK, there is currently one physiotherapist for every 1,136 people compared to Germany where there is one for every 430 people.'

The CSP is urging the government to increase the number of registered physiotherapists by a minimum of 7% annually.

The new analysis also shows that the NHS needs 12,000 more physiotherapists to expand its ability to try and meet demand.

The CSP has lobbied for physiotherapy to be included in the Shortage Occupation List. This addition is key as it will enable businesses and public services to reach talent on a global scale. This should ultimately improve the employability prospects for both domestic and international students.

What is important to note is that significantly more physiotherapists are registered with the HCPC than are employed with the NHS. A growing proportion (approximately 32,000) of physiotherapists work outside the NHS (e.g. in private hospitals, sports clubs or their own private practice), and these are more difficult to track, as the statistics rely on the voluntary registration to the HCPC of physiotherapists. In 2021,

Table 2: Areas of work for physiotherapists

Area	Work
Animal physiotherapist	Supporting animals with the rehabilitation process following a medical operation.
Higher education lecturer	Lecturing on physiotherapy in universities or further education colleges.
Sports therapists	Rehabilitating and providing treatment on sporting injuries, educating athletes and giving advice on prevention.
Acupuncturist	Maintenance of patient health through the process of acupuncture.
Chiropractor	Treating patients through physical manipulation, massage and rehabilitative exercise.
Dance movement psychotherapist	Using dance as a method to develop individuals mentally and emotionally.
Exercise physiologist	Providing scientific support to athletes and sports teams.
Health service manager	Operational responsibility within a hospital, GP surgery or community health service.
Health improvement practitioner	Encouraging lifestyle and behavioural changes to improve overall health and wellbeing.
Osteopath	Treatment of various musculoskeletal health issues.
Personal trainer	Helping others to achieve their fitness goals, more commonly within a gym setting.

60% of CSP members employed by the NHS considered or pursued non-NHS employment within the 12 months prior, while a further 20% actively sought to move out of the NHS. The number of vacancies within the NHS has consequently more than tripled between September 2019 and September 2021.

In the last CSP membership review (2021), there were 74% female to 26% male physiotherapists. Physiotherapists have a relatively young age profile, with 57% of CSP members being under 40 years of age; this is key as it shows a surge in retirement is not expected.

You can maximise your chances of employment by studying for a degree accredited by the CSP and the HCPC and also by being a student member of the CSP.

My main drive for wanting to become an accredited physiotherapist was the desire to help people and provide them with the knowledge of how to better look after their bodies after an injury. I've always been interested in physiology and how the body works and repairs itself after trauma. Being a keen runner who has represented both my school and university in the 800 metres and 1500 metres, I naturally researched my injuries and how I could best avoid repeating them! I always envisaged myself working with athletes or maybe for a professional sports club after completing my BSc in Physiotherapy, but now I'm not so sure. From my placements at the local hospital, through my course, I now have a much wider knowledge of what it means to be a physiotherapist and the varying fields you can work in. The pleasure I have got from working and helping people with long-term disabilities such as cerebral palsy or chronic physical conditions has shown me where my future career lies. I would therefore advise anyone who wants to become a physiotherapist to go into the profession with an open mind and see the discipline as a whole; rather than just focussing on one area that initially appeals to them. Who knows what you may end up doing?

Monica, London South Bank University

To give you an indication of what pay you could be expecting if you joined the physiotherapy profession, starting salaries for qualified physiotherapists (band 5) range from £29,969 to £36,483. Senior physiotherapists can earn between £37,339 and £44,962 (band 6). As a clinical specialist/team leader, you can earn between £46,148 and £52,809 (band 7). Salaries for advanced practice, extended scope or clinical lead physiotherapists range from £53,754 to £60,503 (band 8a). Salaries rise to £85,601 (band 8c) for management roles, such as head of service. For a more detailed breakdown of salaries and bands, please visit: www.nhsbands.co.uk.

As physiotherapists progress in their careers, they are expected to keep up to date with the CPD framework detailed below. As they do this and achieve higher levels of responsibility – and indeed reach team leadership and management roles – they have the opportunity to increase their earnings.

The NHS has a structured tiering of pay grades, and you will need to follow their framework in order to move up the scales. However, private practice is of course different, with remuneration determined by market forces, such as competition and demand. In-house private physiotherapy, such as in sports clubs, for example, will determine the pay scales themselves. However, pay is always determined by experience, and therefore the more emphasis you put on CPD, the quicker you will progress in your career.

Continuing professional development

Throughout their careers, physiotherapists are expected to develop their skills and to keep up to date with developments within the field in a structured and systematic way. This is known as CPD. Physiotherapists are responsible for identifying, planning and recording their own CPD, setting themselves targets and collecting evidence in a portfolio to support their CPD. The process of CPD is summarised in Figure 1.

```
┌─────────────────────────────────────┐
│     Identify areas for improvement    │
└─────────────────────────────────────┘
                  ↓
┌─────────────────────────────────────┐
│      Collect evidence for portfolio   │
└─────────────────────────────────────┘
                  ↓
┌─────────────────────────────────────┐
│           Evaluate outcomes           │
└─────────────────────────────────────┘
                  ↓
┌─────────────────────────────────────┐
│    Activities to achieve these goals  │
└─────────────────────────────────────┘
                  ↓
┌─────────────────────────────────────┐
│             Identify goals            │
└─────────────────────────────────────┘
                  ↓
┌─────────────────────────────────────┐
│            Related courses            │
└─────────────────────────────────────┘
```

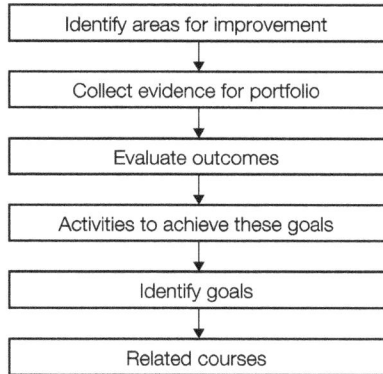

Figure 1: Process of continuing professional development (CPD)

Occupational therapy

While there are a number of differences between physiotherapy and occupational therapy, a lot of similarities are also found. The link is often between dealing with the physical and the mental faculties of a patient in order to ensure their overall rehabilitation. Occupational therapists help people to carry out the tasks and activities that are necessary for them to lead a fulfilling life. These might be work related – helping people with disabilities to cope with their jobs – or they might be everyday things such as cooking, bathing, travelling or socialising. Occupational therapists work in hospitals, for charities and social organisations, in schools and the workplace, in prisons, within the local community and in many other situations. Occupational therapists deal with physical, mental and social needs, for example:

- helping children deal with learning difficulties;
- helping people with mental illness to look after themselves or to be successful in their jobs;
- working with accident victims to enable them to relearn physical tasks;
- advising businesses about how to adapt facilities and premises to enable people with disabilities to cope with their jobs;
- creating rehabilitation programmes for refugees or the homeless.

To practise as an occupational therapist, it is necessary to follow a degree course, either undergraduate or postgraduate, in occupational therapy that has been approved by the HCPC and accredited by the Royal College of Occupational Therapists (RCOT). Graduates seeking international experience may seek a degree that is also approved by the World Federation of Occupational Therapy (WFOT).

Contact details for the RCOT and other useful organisations can be found in Chapter 11.

Case study: Hayden, Senior Physiotherapist at the Queen Elizabeth Hospital, Birmingham

Hayden has always been passionate about pursuing a career in the healthcare sector, driven by his desire to make a meaningful impact on people's lives and further understand the human body. After work experience placements at his local hospital, Hayden found that his true calling lay in physiotherapy, and after numerous years of hard work and dedication, Hayden is now a senior physiotherapist at the Queen Elizabeth Hospital, Birmingham.

'Like many others who pursued studying physiotherapy, my initial interest came from a combination of interest in sports, biology and the workings of the human body. My initial thoughts regarding career choices were pointing me in the direction of healthcare, and I gained some work experience initially within the radiology and oncology departments at my local hospital. Following this, by gaining some understanding of the different roles available in health care and then seeing first-hand physios working in the rehabilitation of my family members, physiotherapy appeared to be a career that would offer great reward and satisfaction and would suit my preference for a more practical and active style of working.

'As I began to research more into physiotherapy, I realised there were far more components and aspects of the job beyond the traditional view of physios working in sports and rehabilitation. I became more aware of the roles of physiotherapists in working with a range of neurological, respiratory and musculoskeletal conditions across a range of settings in health care and private practice.

'I therefore sought to gain as much work experience within these different areas as I could. I was fortunate to arrange time shadowing a community neurophysiotherapist working in the rehabilitation of patients with a range of neurological conditions, such as stroke, multiple sclerosis and Parkinson's disease. While this was very eye-opening and contrasted sharply with my initial expectations of physiotherapy, it showed me the hugely important role that physios can play in people's lives and the opportunity for great satisfaction within the job role. Through contacts made during this work experience, I began volunteering with a local exercise group run for patients with multiple sclerosis, which enabled me to get more hands-on experience of helping patients with this condition.

'I gained this experience while I completed A levels in Biology, which was essential for the course, as well as Chemistry and History.

'I gained further experience by applying to the work experience departments at all of my local hospitals, which enabled me to shadow physiotherapists working in areas of trauma and respiratory physiotherapy, which again showed me the varying nature of the role. I tried to be proactive in contacting many local private physiotherapists and found that many were very welcoming in allowing me to shadow their work in treating patients with a range of musculoskeletal injuries and conditions. I also arranged time shadowing physiotherapists working within a school for children with a range of disabilities, allowing me to see a range of methods physiotherapists can use to overcome significant physical and psychological barriers, while also keeping treatment fun and engaging.

'I feel that this variety of work experience was hugely beneficial in my application process for universities and gave me a range of experiences to discuss in subsequent interviews. I would advise anyone considering a career in physiotherapy to be as proactive in gaining as much experience as possible, to enable them to fully understand the roles that they are applying for, as well as strengthening their application.

'The application process after the personal statement submission varied across different universities. Some required group interviews, where certain tasks would be set to complete as a group, and most required an individual interview. The interview panels are particularly interested in ensuring applicants have a good understanding of the profession and the different areas involved. They will be interested in hearing about your previous experiences and what you have learned from them. The interview is an opportunity to show skills in communication and problem-solving and qualities of compassion and enthusiasm.

'The Physiotherapy course itself will also vary between universities in terms of course structure, teaching styles and opportunities for experience in clinical placements. It is important to therefore research and explore the universities before applying in order to find a course that most suits you.

'I completed my training at Plymouth University, and I am now working in a senior physiotherapy role within an NHS hospital. The course requires a lot of learning and hard work but is worth it in progressing into a line of work that is interesting, massively varied and rewarding.'

Hayden went to the University of Plymouth after achieving AAA in his A levels.

2 | Strengthen your core
Physiotherapy courses: What to expect

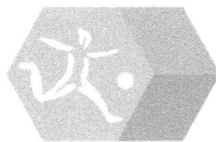

This chapter deals with the types of courses that you can expect at university. It looks at the typical structure of a BSc as well as the different teaching approaches you might find. It also discusses courses in Scotland, Wales and Northern Ireland and the differences in course style, as well as MSc (pre-registration) courses. It is useful to note that these are guidelines and that courses can vary between universities, so make sure you research the available courses properly.

In the UK, as mentioned in the previous chapter, a physiotherapist requires a degree from a CSP/HCPC-accredited course in order to practise with confidence. In turn, if you practise in the UK, you are required by law to be registered with the HCPC. An accredited three-year degree will allow you to register with the HCPC and CSP after graduation. All undergraduate Physiotherapy degree programmes in the UK at mainstream universities are accredited by the CSP.

Physiotherapy is a very competitive course, and, as such, the entry levels will be set higher than the minimum. For many universities, there are no prescribed A levels that you should take, unlike for medicine, although some universities do request biology (or human biology). Others might request one or two scientific subjects more broadly, so you should still carefully consider what to study for your A levels; for example, psychology would be better as a third subject than film studies. Physical education or sports science is often listed as a requirement, either as an alternative to or in addition to biology. Top GCSE grades (7–9/A–B) are highly desirable, and you will need to achieve competitive A level results, usually in the A–B grade bracket, depending on the academic establishment, with AAA–ABB being a typical offer. However, always bear in mind that entry requirements from universities are the minimum. A lot of people will be applying with higher predicted grades, and there is also much more to the application than academic achievement, which we will discuss later in the book.

The key for now is to check each individual university's website in order to find out the details you require.

Typical course structure

In accordance with good practice set out by the HCPC, all UK Physiotherapy courses are revalidated every five to seven years. While all Physiotherapy courses contain many common elements, there are significant differences in the structure of courses, in the course content, in the way in which the practical and patient-contact elements are arranged and in the styles of assessment. You should investigate this thoroughly by reading prospectuses and looking at the physiotherapy departments' websites in order to find out which ones will suit you best.

In a continuing move towards the development of physiotherapy in the community and the focus on prevention, many universities have adjusted their courses to reflect this and to help students meet the changing state of the NHS and be able to work successfully within it.

Example course structure: Brunel University of London

Year 1

- Anatomy 1: Lower Quadrant
- Principles of Rehabilitation
- Systems of Physiology and Pathophysiology
- Anatomy 2: Upper Quadrant
- Person Centred Healthcare and Leadership 1
- Musculoskeletal Lower Quadrant 1
- Respiratory

Year 2

- Musculoskeletal 2: Upper Quadrant
- Practice Placements 1 and 2
- Mandatory Clinical Training
- Person Centred Healthcare and Leadership 2
- Neurorehabilitation
- Cardiovascular Health
- Research Methods

Year 3

- Critical Care
- Practice Placement 3, 4 and 5
- Health Across the Lifespan
- Transition to Professional Practice
- Research Proposals

Source: www.brunel.ac.uk/study/undergraduate/physiotherapy-bsc.
Reprinted with kind permission of Brunel University of London.

Research dissertation

There will be continuing modules in research alongside the clinical placements. Evidence-based practice is essential in physiotherapy; therefore, students need to learn how to carry out research as well as how to use existing research. For all honours degrees, this is a major component of the course in the second and third years, and there is a focus towards a research dissertation that will be submitted in the final year. This part of the course enables you to manage and organise a research project. You will choose an area of interest in the field of physiotherapy. Here you will consolidate and develop your analytical skills and critically evaluate found evidence. Most dissertations will be around 10,000 words in length.

Elective clinical placement

At the end of the third year, there may be an elective clinical placement. You will choose the speciality in which you wish to work and arrange the placement yourself. Many students choose to work abroad or in areas of healthcare not previously encountered in their own clinical education.

Be aware of the different teaching styles of the courses and refer to the universities' websites to find all the information. Some courses are modular, some have a lot of emphasis on clinical teaching and others are more theoretical. You need to find out which courses best suit your needs, offer you the opportunities you seek and will help you flourish.

Teaching styles

These will be different, depending on the instructor and the course material; however, they can broadly be split into the following types:

- **Interactive.** An interactive style is what the name implies, with discussions, Q&A sessions and presentations. This style suits those who have already absorbed the facts, and students will pursue independent research and build on this through the practical aspects of the course.
- **Lecture.** A lecture is useful for providing a lot of facts in one session, which will then be researched further outside the course. This implies extra reading to supplement what you have been taught.
- **Problem-based learning (PBL).** This is student-centred learning where you will learn about topics by looking at multifaceted and realistic problems. You will work in groups and identify what you know, what you need to know and how you will find the information

necessary for solving the problems. The instructor will ask questions and provide resources to lead you to the right answers. However, you must figure the answers out for yourself.

* **Practice-based professional learning (PBPL).** This style requires a level of professional practice in order to fully understand the course. It is in contrast to theory-led learning and is directly related to the practical aspects of the course. It is a new style of learning and is prevalent in the newer universities.

You should look on the websites for the individual universities to find out which teaching styles they use. See Chapter 11 for university contact details.

Courses in Scotland

There are three universities in Scotland where you can study physiotherapy:

1.   Queen Margaret University, Edinburgh;
2.   Glasgow Caledonian University;
3.   Robert Gordon University, Aberdeen.

The courses are four years full time, rather than three years full time as in England. The courses have a strong clinical bias with work placements, and you are required to complete an honours project in your fourth year.

It is also possible to take a two-year MSc in Physiotherapy pre-registration course after taking a different degree. This allows students another opportunity to study physiotherapy after having studied in a different but scientifically related discipline.

The section below summarises the options on offer on the Scottish courses so that you can see the different approaches of a Scottish university. Apart from the length of the course, you will see that they are not wholly dissimilar to the English courses.

Queen Margaret University

Year 1 is spent learning the basic and applied sciences needed for physiotherapy. Year 2 begins to focus more on cardiorespiratory, musculoskeletal and neurological physiotherapy. Year 3 will develop skills in people management and understanding of health education. In the final year, you will complete a research project with the support of a project supervisor while also consolidating knowledge and skills with practice-based learning placements.

Part of your learning will be alongside an experienced, registered physiotherapist working with patients, carers and/or families. It is important to work with other health and social care professionals to see the role each plays in a patient's care. Practice-based learning is employed in settings around Scotland; this is funded by you. It may be possible to take one optional practice-based placement overseas.

Glasgow Caledonian University

The aim of this course is to give you the professional and academic knowledge and skills needed to manage individual patients. This course promotes your critical analysis skills, which you will have to use to justify and evaluate evidence in your practical work. This will be particularly relevant in your honours project in the fourth year. You will also visit clinical simulation labs, take field trips, have educational placements and use e-learning. There is scope to gain experience in a placement in the UK or abroad. Students will undertake at least 1,000 hours of supervised practice placement experience during their study. Healthy lifestyles and physical activity are promoted heavily in this course, and placements play a big part in supplementing your learning.

Robert Gordon University

A very modern course, this is designed to help you 'meet the demands of the rapidly changing health sector'. The clinical placement is of primary importance, as it gives you the 'real' experiences that will ensure your professional credibility.

This is very much a practical course, with a high proportion of practical assessment within the first two years. The faculty building offers state-of-the-art teaching and clinical skills facilities. You will use practical therapy rooms and a human performance laboratory. There is also a 'sophisticated three-dimensional motion analysis system' that will allow you to see in action what it is you are being taught. There is also a unique, computerised 'METIMan' in the clinical skills area where you will be able to practise before going into a real-life setting.

The final year will put most emphasis on evaluation and research skills and two final clinical placements to refine the necessary techniques required for the profession.

Courses in Wales

The section below summarises the three-year, full-time options on offer at Cardiff University and Wrexham University. If you study physiotherapy at either of these universities and agree to work in Wales for two years upon completion of your studies, you may be eligible to receive the NHS Wales Bursary – this means that your tuition fees are paid, and you will receive an annual £1,000 grant payment.

Alternatively, the University of South Wales offers a part-time Physiotherapy degree of four years or longer.

Cardiff University

The department is over 100 years old and offers a CSP-accredited degree over three years. The diversity and complexity of the profession are mirrored in the theory and practice elements of this course. It combines university lectures with seven four-week placements spread across Years 2 and 3. You will learn from both academic and clinical physiotherapists, creating a holistic approach. Students gain experience in all of the core areas of the profession. Placements take place around Wales but may also be arranged in other locations in order to maintain high standards. The university endeavours to provide students with extracurricular opportunities, most notably volunteering their skills to support the annual Cardiff Half Marathon.

Wrexham University

Studies during the first year lay down the foundational knowledge and skills of problem-solving and clinical reasoning. A four-week placement provides an opportunity for students to reflect on the learning and prepare for the level 5 placement experience. Year 2 develops knowledge and skills in greater depth through studies in cardiorespiratory, neurology and the spine and provides a seven-week placement to consolidate the skills and knowledge from Years 1 and 2. Year 3 offers increased opportunities for independent learning and self-reflection in preparation for employment.

Courses in Northern Ireland

The section below summarises the options on offer at the University of Ulster.

University of Ulster

In Northern Ireland, there is one principal university recognised by the CSP teaching the Physiotherapy course, the University of Ulster. As in the other universities discussed above, there is a split between theory and practice, but a large emphasis is placed on practice-based learning. Applicants will also be video interviewed as part of the admissions process.

In Years 1 and 2 of the programme, you will usually take at least six modules, including inter-professional modules. In the final year, students will undertake either an investigative project or a dissertation. A feature of this course is the integration of theory and practice; participation is expected from everyone, and peer examination is used as a testing device. The University of Ulster uses practice-based learning. Beginning in your first year, you will take part in five clinical placements during the course, totalling 30 weeks, to help confirm your learning.

MSc (pre-registration) course

This is different from the postgraduate MSc in Physiotherapy, which is for students who have already trained as physiotherapists and now want to specialise. The MSc (pre-registration) course, for students who have not yet trained in physiotherapy, is a two-year, full-time qualifying programme for graduates with a suitable and relevant first degree. This would usually be a scientific subject based around biology, that is, biology, behavioural science, physiology and so on. (This course is arguably even more competitive than the BSc entry because of both the number of applicants and the demands placed on you.)

The course aims to give students with the necessary skills a second opportunity to take on evidence-based physiotherapy programmes with a variety of patients. A large emphasis is placed on the implementation of research and auditing programmes. This course is accredited by the CSP and the HCPC.

Course overview

The course is divided between research and clinical placements. A large emphasis is placed on the latter, which is typically arranged over six modules with over 1,000 hours of study. Students will treat patients and watch professionals in different settings, from in-house to home visits. There are three core areas: the management of neurological, cardiopulmonary and neuromusculoskeletal dysfunctions, with knowledge from the biomedical and psychosocial sciences recruited as required.

First year

The first year develops practice and reasoning in the core areas of practice. Evaluation and critical analysis are key to development in terms of physiotherapeutic concepts. In the last part of the year, students begin their research project.

Second year

The clinical modules and research project continue during the second year. There will also be work on an Advancing Physiotherapy module, which addresses other approaches to the management of physiotherapy.

Practice placements

These are a key factor in the education of a physiotherapist and will take place over the two-year study, usually occupying 1,000 hours in total. You will normally be seconded to a range of diverse and exciting placements, where you will gain a variety of experience with numerous client groups under the guidance of skilled clinicians. Each student will gain experience in physiotherapy within various placement settings.

3| Pulled in every direction
Work experience

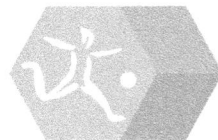

According to the Chartered Society of Physiotherapy:

Gaining relevant work experience will help your application because admissions tutors are looking for evidence that you have an understanding of the profession and can communicate well with people, of all ages or backgrounds. However, work experience can be difficult to organise because of current training pressures on practices and relevant hospital departments. If you cannot work or volunteer directly with physios, work experience in any aspect of healthcare will be useful to you. Organisations you could approach include: your local hospital, sports clinics, football clubs, schools or units for children or adults with disabilities, nursing homes, voluntary organisations (e.g. Red Cross Association, St John's Ambulance Society, MS Society).

Information taken from the Chartered Society of Physiotherapy (www.csp.org.uk), with kind permission from the CSP

Work experience is important for gaining entry into physiotherapy, as it provides first-hand insight into the profession, demonstrates commitment to the course and helps develop essential skills like communication, empathy and problem-solving. It allows applicants to confirm their career choice, understand the challenges of the role and gain exposure to professional conduct in clinical settings. It is your introduction to the profession at first-hand and evidence that you have worked with people in the community. For example, St George's stresses they require students 'to have an understanding of the realities of working as a healthcare professional and show they have the necessary skills and attributes for their chosen career'. They go on to advise online resources as an alternative way to seek this insight.

If you are very lucky (and very determined), you may be able to get a paid job in an NHS hospital as a physiotherapy assistant. However, because of school or college commitments, this is usually only possible during a gap year. It is more likely that you will have to settle for an unpaid volunteer position either on a part-time basis (on weekends or in the evenings) or for a short period of time in the school holidays.

Even before the pandemic, training pressures on hospital-based physiotherapy departments were making it difficult to get any relevant work experience; these pressures are even greater now, so anything within a health-related or care field will be very useful.

If you are unable to arrange any of the above, you should try to shadow a physiotherapist for a day or two and supplement this with a volunteer job in another caring environment, such as a hospice or special school. There are also a growing number of medicine-related summer schools and experiences that provide demonstrable insight into the profession.

Be fastidious in your investigation of how much work experience is required per institution. The universities' own websites are your starting place, followed by contacting the university directly if it does not publish the information.

Length of time

While there are no rules about the minimum length of time that you should spend doing work experience, volunteer work or work-shadowing, as a general rule, those candidates who can demonstrate commitment by doing something on a regular basis throughout the year or who have spent at least two weeks in a hospital environment are likely to be in the strongest position. The current economic climate may require you to think outside the box. For example, you could volunteer in a care home or on a children's ward in a hospital and watch the nurses and physiotherapists there. You can also chat with physiotherapists or go to physiotherapy appointments with friends or relatives.

> Get as much experience as you can – it doesn't just have to be as a physiotherapy assistant. Be determined: there is always a way to get in if you really want to.
>
> Katherine, University of Hertfordshire

Hospitals will often provide an opportunity for students to do a one-day work experience, and you should contact them directly regarding these opportunities.

Some schools operate schemes where they arrange work experience for you. This saves you the hard work of contacting hospitals or clinics, but the drawback is that you will be unable to impress the selectors with your dynamism and determination because you will not be able to say, 'I arranged my work experience myself'.

How to apply

If your school does not operate such a scheme, you have two options: to use any contacts that your family or friends have or to approach local hospitals. To do the latter, you need to get the names and addresses of local hospitals with physiotherapy departments and physiotherapy clinics from the internet. You should send an email to the hospital or clinic and include the name of a referee – someone who can vouch for your interest in physiotherapy as well as for your reliability. Your careers teacher, housemaster or housemistress, or form teacher would be ideal. An example of a suitable email is given below.

From: Rachel Thompson
To: oakparkcare@wakeford.gov.uk
Subject: Volunteering

Dear Sir/Madam,

I am a Year 12, A level student interested in pursuing a career in physiotherapy. I plan to apply to study physiotherapy at university and am looking to gain as much experience as possible in this field. My interest in physiotherapy was sparked after attending an appointment with my grandmother after she sustained an injury. I was fascinated by the process of her recovery, and though I have always enjoyed studying the sciences, I had never been inspired by a specific career before. I have heard that you are looking for volunteers, and I would be delighted if you would consider me for a role. I am available in the evenings and on weekends, so please let me know if you think this would be suitable for you. I am more than happy to discuss this further in person, and if you require a reference, please contact my form tutor:
Mr Shaw
Featherstone Academy
Wakeford
WF8 7BY
a.shaw@featherstone.ac.uk

Thank you for your consideration.

Yours sincerely,
Rachel Thompson

When applying for work experience, you will need to create a CV for the potential employers to get an idea of your skills and education. This is basically a summary of what you have done so far in your life to date. Within the CV will be your up-to-date contact details, educational qualifications and, of course, any previous work experience. Please see the sample CV opposite.

CV

Personal details

Richard Hall
16 St Mary's Avenue
Peterborough
PE21 5TU
01733 523559
r.a.hall@zmail.co.uk

Education and qualifications

2024–present: Kingswood High School, Peterborough
A levels: Biology, Chemistry, Physical Education
GCSEs (June 2024): Mathematics 8, English Language 8, English
Literature 9, History 7, Physics 8, Chemistry 8, Biology 9, Spanish 7

Work experience

July 2024–present: High Street Book Shop, Peterborough
Responsible for till work, replenishing stock from the storeroom,
stocktaking and general duties.
October 2023–June 2024: Sales Assistant at local superstore
Duties included helping customers with their questions and needs. Also
stocking shelves and some cashier work.

Skills

Languages – good written and spoken Spanish
Computing – competent in Word and Excel

Interests

I'm a keen cricket player and represent my local first team. I'm also
interested in world cinema and am a member of the school film club.

References

Mr J. Featherstone
Head of Sixth Form
Kingswood High School
Peterborough
j.featherstone@kingswood.ac.uk
Mrs K. Blake
Eastman's Bookshop
High Street
Peterborough
k.l.blake@eastmans.co.uk

As well as helping you to decide whether you are serious about physiotherapy and adding weight to your application, work experience is useful because you may be able to get one of the people you work with to give you a reference, which you could send in support of your UCAS application or produce at your interview.

Work experience in Wales

While you are at school or college, NHS Wales Informatics Service will support and help you decide on your next career move by offering work experience placements for one to 10 weeks. However, work placements can be hard to come by. Gaining work experience in NHS Wales can be quite challenging for individuals under 18. However, students aged 14–18 who are in full-time education may have opportunities for work experience. To find the latest updates on available placements, you can visit the following website. www.cavuhb.nhs.wales/our-services/work -experience/.

Cardiff University and Wrexham University therefore do not stipulate work experience as being essential but do want to see that applicants have spoken to physiotherapists or physiotherapy students, that they have looked at physiotherapy-related publications and they have contacted the CSP (which has a pretty comprehensive careers page).

Things to look out for during work experience

The variety of treatments available to patients

Make sure that you know what you are observing. Ask the physiotherapist or nurse for the technical names of the procedures that you see and for information on the techniques and equipment used. Ask about the advantages and disadvantages of different types of treatments and in what situations they are used. Keep a diary of what you saw on a day-to-day basis, so that you can use it to revise prior to an interview. There are a number of websites that provide detailed information on medical conditions and treatments, and you could add further detail to your diary using one of these. See the list of 'Useful websites' at the end of the book.

Working as a physiotherapist

Ask the physiotherapist about his or her work life. Find out about the hours, the pay, the demands of the job and the career options open to physiotherapists. Find out what the physiotherapists like about the job and what they dislike.

Case study: Jessie, second-year student at the University of Liverpool

'Studying at Liverpool University for physiotherapy has been an amazing experience so far and one of my proudest achievements. Although coming straight from sixth form made me apprehensive initially, with perhaps less clinical experience than more mature students, I soon realised this wasn't a disadvantage. As a small cohort you get to know other students well and share experiences, while the lecturers encourage you and support you in the whole university experience.

'Many of our tutors are currently still employed in private or public practices, and they have provided opportunities and ideas for us outside of university lectures. Some of us have volunteered with local charities and hospitals, while external talks have provided an insight into different areas you can specialise in as a physiotherapist.

'We had about eight weeks out on practice in our first year of the course, with one week of this being an observational placement, which provided us the opportunity to put into perspective our knowledge at an early stage. All the other placements are six weeks at a time, divided evenly over the next few years to get over 1,000 hours on placement and become qualified. The university tries to get you a wide range of placements, such as respiratory, neurological, community and out-patient placements soon after covering those modules at university.

'Now in Year 2 of my Physiotherapy course the intensity of study and research has increased. An average day starts at 10am and finishes at 5pm, with lunch and breaks. The day is usually split into two hours of theory in the morning, then putting this into "hands-on" practice in the afternoon, using each other as models, so you soon become comfortable with each other. There is always more work to do outside lecture hours, but this is manageable and there is time allocated for this.

'The physiotherapy lectures are mostly based on the campus. We have breaks between lectures and it's a good idea to consolidate our learning at the library; it has all of the resources you can wish for, and is a great place to study. Each project or assessment is different on the course, and so caters for all types of learners and enables a large range of skills for when we go out on placement.

'I'd say my most enjoyable side of physiotherapy so far is the time I spend with patients, as each assessment is different and to hear their stories of their accidents or condition is fascinating. I'm looking forward to studying outpatients and seeing how different this will be from what we have done before. After my completion of the course I have the next goal of securing a rotational band 5 physiotherapy position, which will lead on to securing a speciality area where I can begin my career and become the best physio I can be!'

Tips for work experience

- Dress as the physiotherapists dress: be clean, tidy and reasonably formal. There are no strict rules here. You should dress professionally – some wear a shirt and tie, in sports physiotherapy you might wear shorts and a polo shirt, and hospitals have their own specific uniforms. Use your common sense!
- Research the company that you are being interviewed by. What are their products? What is their history?
- Expand on your key skills and attributes.
- What times and dates are you available to work for them.
- Offer to help the physiotherapist or the nurses with routine tasks.
- Show an interest in everything that is going on around you.

While my grandmother was in a care home in Leicestershire I enquired with the NHS management at the home if there was an opportunity for me to volunteer and help with the patients' physiotherapy. I was delighted that they agreed and I was able to help for about four hours per week. This experience showed me that I did indeed want to forge a career in physiotherapy. It also gave me great satisfaction: I was doing a job (even though voluntary) that had a massive positive effect on the people I was helping, and I gained so much valuable experience from the qualified team of physiotherapists who worked there.

Ellen, University of Manchester

Discussing your work experience at interview

If you are fortunate enough to be called for an interview, then you can expect to discuss your work experience. It is a great way for an interviewer to get to know you and find out more about your research. It would be a good idea to ask the employers where you volunteered to write a reference for you.

So, remember these golden points about the purpose of work experience to mention in the interview:

- confirmed your choice of study;
- important for learning skills, which include teamwork, independence, administration and so on;
- working hours;
- care-based profession.

All the time with work experience, keep remembering what you are learning from the experience. The weakest applications are the ones that just mention work experience for the sake of it. There is nothing worse than a personal statement or interview with just a catalogue of work experiences but no substance behind them, as that is pure vanity. Work experience will form the basis of your discussions. Make some notes about what you learn as you go and take those notes with you on the day of your interview.

4 | On the rack/under observation
The UCAS application

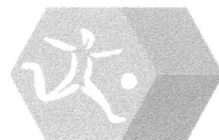

In order to gain a place at university, you have to submit a UCAS application. Before you do this, however, you need to be sure that you have investigated physiotherapy as thoroughly as you can. You need to do this for two reasons:

1. You must be sure that physiotherapy is the right career for you.
2. You must demonstrate to the university admissions tutors that you are aware of the demands of the profession.

With so many applicants for every university place, the selectors need to be sure that they do not 'waste' a place on someone who will then drop out of the course or the profession. The rate of offers for UK school leavers (approximate) varies, depending on the institution; for example, Birmingham has one in five students receiving offers, whereas Southampton, at the opposite end of the scale, has three in 20 students receiving offers. For this reason, your application has to be very convincing. Most people's exposure to physiotherapy is limited, and so you need to investigate the profession in depth.

Choice of university

Once you have completed your work experience and are sure that you want to be a physiotherapist, you need to research your choice of university. There are various factors that you should take into account:

- the type of course;
- the entrance requirements;
- location;
- whether you will be taught alongside students on other healthcare courses such as radiology, nursing, occupational therapy or podiatry.

Research

The first thing to do is to get hold of the prospectuses. If your school does not have spare copies, telephone the universities; they will send you a prospectus free of charge. You can also order these online, which is the quickest way of doing this, and most have a downloadable PDF for you to look at too. All universities have very informative websites that carry extra information on admissions policies.

> **TIP!**
>
> Do not simply select your universities because someone tells you that they have good reputations or that they are easier to get into, because you will be spending the next three or four years of your life at one of them, and if you do not like the place, you are unlikely to last the course.

Apart from talking to current or former physiotherapy students or careers advisers, there are a number of other sources of information. The *Guardian* newspaper publishes its own league table of universities (www.theguardian.com/education/universityguide), ranked by a total score that combines the university's teaching assessment, a 'value added' score based on the class of degree obtained compared with A level (or equivalent) grades, spending on facilities and materials, student/staff ratios, job prospects and entrance requirements. *The Times* also compiles its own table, but this can only be accessed through a subscription payment. The Complete University Guide league table can be found at www.thecompleteuniversityguide.co.uk /league-tables/rankings.

Other websites that are worth checking are the National Student Survey (www.thestudentsurvey.com), which gives existing undergraduate students a platform to share their experiences of colleges, courses and teaching, and Discover Uni (www.discoveruni.gov.uk), which 'includes official statistics about higher education courses taken from national surveys and data collected from universities and colleges about their students'.

Of course, league tables tell you only a small part of the whole story, and anyone who makes their choices solely on this basis without visiting the universities or reading the prospectuses is taking a serious risk.

Open days

Once you have narrowed down the number of universities to, say, seven or eight, you should try to visit them in order to get a better idea of what studying there would be like. Your school careers department will have details of open days (or you could telephone the universities directly).

Equally, you can look on the websites and, for those that have the facility, use their online booking system for open days. Open days always get fully booked, so the earlier you do it, the better. Some universities will arrange for you to be shown around at other times of the year as well.

Going to open days also gives you the opportunity to ask an admissions tutor any questions that you might have about the university generally, such as about sporting activities, societies or accommodation. You should go with a list of questions and show yourself to be proactive. After all, you would not go shopping for clothes without trying them on! Details can be found on the university websites.

Several universities began to run online open days or seminars during the pandemic, and most still offer virtual solutions in some capacity, such as virtual campus tours, live webinars and on-demand information videos. Many universities also now offer alumni chat functions on their websites, which can provide you with a different perspective on university life. While online events are more effective when it comes to the time and cost of travelling, it can be more difficult to gauge the feel of a campus, and it's not so easy to ask questions.

Try to go to as many open days as you can, providing you are allowed to by your school. If you cannot attend the open day, go and have a look on another day and email any questions you have to the admissions tutor. Do not ask questions to which you can find answers for yourself on the website, such as 'What is the grade requirement?'; this does not show you to be proactive, just lazy. Ask for details, not generics.

Entrance requirements

Entrance requirements vary from university to university, but a 'standard' offer might ask for a minimum of ABB, with Russell Group universities often asking for AAB. The offer will probably specify that biology must be studied at A level, along with one other science. A* grades are not usually asked for but do represent higher points. It is most common that you will be given an offer based on getting three grades, as opposed to points. It is worthwhile checking your offer conditions when they come through to see whether points are also accepted; offers expressed as points are usually a minimum of 128 points from three A levels or equivalent.

You should also check the university prospectuses for details of A level requirements. Some universities, for example, may specify that they require one of the subjects to be an arts subject or humanity rather than them all being science subjects or mathematics.

If we take the University of Brighton's entry requirements as an example, then you will need to obtain ABB (128 UCAS points), including Biology, Human Biology or PE.

Other common qualifications that can also gain you access to courses are listed below:

Access to HE Diploma

A QAA-recognised Access to Science course which must include biological science. Pass with a minimum of 60 credits, 45 of which must be at level 3 (at least 30 distinctions and 15 merits).

BTEC Extended Diploma

DDM, and an A level in Biology or Human Biology at grade B.

BTEC Higher National Diploma

DD in the BTEC National Diploma, to normally be accompanied by an A grade in a Science A level.

Cambridge Pre-U

Combinations of three subjects allowed, normally including Biology or PE, usually looking towards a D3/M1 or higher.

International Baccalaureate

32 points, with a 6 in Biology at Higher level.

Irish Leaving Certificate

Typically H2, H3, H3, H3, H3, which must include Biology and English.

Scottish qualifications

Typically three As and two Bs at higher level, which must include Biology and English.

T levels

D in the Health, Healthcare Science or Science T level; other T levels are not accepted.

The UCAS Tariff

The UCAS Tariff is the system for allocating points to qualifications used for entry to higher education. However, what UCAS does say is that a lot of universities do not use the Tariff system and rely solely on grade offers, so do not worry unnecessarily about this Tariff; instead, focus on getting those grades.

A conversion chart for A level grades to UCAS Tariff points is given in Table 3, overleaf.

Table 3: UCAS Tariff conversion chart

	UCAS Tariff
A level grade A*	56
A level grade A	48
A level grade B	40
A level grade C	32
A level grade D	24
A level grade E	16

We acknowledge UCAS's contribution of this information.

Your choices

There are five spaces in the UCAS application, all of which may be used for Physiotherapy courses. (In contrast, students applying for medicine, dentistry or veterinary science may use only four of their five choices for such courses.) You do not have to fill all five spaces with Physiotherapy courses. The key point to note here is that universities cannot see who else you have applied to, and the order on the form is alphabetical, so you do not have to know your order from the outset. Only once you have got your offers will you put down Conditional Firm and Conditional Insurance. Therefore, you are allowed to apply for a mixture of Physiotherapy courses and non-Physiotherapy courses or to leave spaces blank. Thus, the important part is the personal statement, as it must be written to reflect the course you are applying for at university. As all the courses have to be reflected in the same personal statement, they all have to be broadly similar in order to be sure that the personal statement can be tailored to each of your five choices without any ambiguity in terms of what you are applying for.

If you are worried that you might not be offered a place to study physiotherapy and you would consider other courses, you might want to put down four Physiotherapy courses and one other course. The one non-Physiotherapy course should be related to physiotherapy, either directly (occupational therapy, podiatry) or in a related discipline such as human biology or physiology. Other courses, such as Radiology or Nursing, are not related, for example. You should not enter fewer than four Physiotherapy courses in the application – if you do, you are unlikely to convince the selectors that you are genuinely committed, not because they will know what other courses you have applied for, but because your personal statement will not reflect physiotherapy as much as it should.

> **TIP!**
>
> Applying for other courses, such as medicine or veterinary science, alongside your Physiotherapy course should be avoided. It will be clear to the admissions tutors from your personal statement that you are not 100% committed to physiotherapy and therefore your application will not be taken seriously. Also, it will cause you problems writing your personal statement when giving reasons for your desire to have a career in physiotherapy.

If you decide that you would be happy to accept an alternative if your application for physiotherapy is unsuccessful, by all means choose another course, as long as you feel able to justify the choice at the interview. However, our advice is to apply only to Physiotherapy courses because:

- The way you write the personal statement should demonstrate to the selectors that you are committed to becoming a physiotherapist.
- You do not run the risk of feeling obliged to accept a place on a course that, at heart, you do not wish to take. If you are unsuccessful in your initial application for physiotherapy, you may be able to gain a place through UCAS Extra or Clearing, if you have accepted no alternative offers.
- The more places you apply to, the more chances you are giving yourself.

Once you have made your final choices, make sure that you have entered the details into the application correctly. More advice on this can be found in *How to Complete Your UCAS Application* (Trotman Education).

When choosing your universities, I found it helpful in my decision making to visit each one. You can get a sense of the university as well as the city or town itself. Open days at universities are so beneficial as the course you are thinking of applying for is explained to you by the department itself. This is the main reason I chose to come to Birmingham to study. The facilities and teaching staff were very impressive and engaging, and their range of course subjects was outstanding. Work placements throughout the study period at Birmingham were impressive thanks to it being a huge, vibrant city with so many differing opportunities. Their employment rates for graduating students was the highest out of my other choices also.

Jonathan, Birmingham

The UCAS application form

UCAS Hub (previously known as UCAS Track) is UCAS's online applications system, which you can use to register and apply to your university choices. The UCAS application is made up of several important sections. The form is straightforward, but it does take time to fill in, so it is important not rush it, as that is when you make mistakes. The sections are as follows:

Personal details: basic information – name, age, title and gender.

Nationality: birthplace and nationality.

Where you live: current address.

Contact details: email and telephone number.

Supporting information: anything universities and providers may need to know to understand what support you might require during your studies.

English language skills: to determine whether English is your first language.

Finance and funding: details of who is paying your tuition fees.

Education: past exam results, information about previous and current schools/colleges, as well as upcoming examinations.

Employment: this is only for paid work, not for any work experience – you should include the employer's name and address.

Extra Activities: any additional activities you wish to include, such as Summer Schools or Open Days you attended.

Personal statement: personal statements are transitioning from a single long text to three distinct sections, each addressing a specific question to help students focus their responses. Each section will require a minimum of 350 characters, with a clearly visible character limit and overall counter to guide students as they write. The updated submission page will also include helpful tips and guidance for each question.

The new questions are:

- Why do you want to study this course or subject?
- How have your qualifications and studies helped you to prepare for this course or subject?
- What else have you done to prepare outside of education, and why are these experiences useful?

The personal statement will still be 4,000 characters in total (including spaces).

Importantly, it should include details of your work experience as the main section. Remember, this is not an essay. Do not use anyone else's words for your personal statement – remember that UCAS has software that will detect this. Check what you have written for accuracy of spelling, punctuation and grammar. Do not be too emphatic – let the content be what will impress an admissions tutor, not your ability to use synonyms (see Chapter 5).

Choices: your five researched university choices

Reference: this is very important. If you are applying through a school, your tutor will write a statement supporting your application and endorsing your potential for the course. Every school has its own guidelines, but in general, the reference should comment on your skills, your abilities and your academic results to date; provide the reasons for any poor results and an explanation of what is being done to rectify this and also a recommendation to the university of you as a student. If you are applying as an independent candidate, you will need to find an academic or professional referee who will follow these guidelines and seek references from other sources to bolster their reference. Referees should read the 'Advisers' section on the website.

Do not rush the application. Take your time and pay attention to the details. Make sure that you have used the correct course and institution codes. Check that you have entered the correct examination boards for your subjects and that all of the dates are accurate. Ensure accuracy throughout the form. Do not miss the deadline, which is usually in the middle of January.

For physiotherapy, the following should also be your guide.

Application checklist:

- At least two weeks of NHS work-shadowing;
- Voluntary work;
- Right GCSE subjects and grades;
- Right A level subjects;
- On target for required grades;
- Looked at all the universities' prospectuses;
- Open days;
- Minimum of four physiotherapy choices in the UCAS application;
- Personal statement demonstrates commitment, research, personal qualities, communication skills and manual dexterity.

Making your application stand out

When your UCAS application is received by the university, it will not be on its own but in a batch of, possibly, several hundred. The selectors will have to consider it, along with the others, in between the demands of their 'real' jobs. If your application is uninteresting, lacking evidence of real commitment to physiotherapy or badly worded, it will be put on the reject pile.

Interviews are an essential part of the UCAS process for physiotherapy. You can be called for an interview only on the basis of your UCAS application. The selectors will not know about the things that you have forgotten to say, and they can get an impression of you only from what is in the application. We have come across too many good students who never got an interview simply because they did not think about the UCAS application; they relied on the hope that the selectors would somehow see through the words and get an instinctive feeling about them. The following sections will tell you more about what the selectors are looking for and how you can avoid common mistakes. Before looking at how the selectors go about deciding whom to call for an interview, however, there are a number of important things that you need to think about.

> *The best thing about candidates is that they are all different. They are all unique. Therefore our advice is clear; don't write as though you are the same as everyone else. Find the things that are personal to you, your motivations, your values and translate them into your writing. This is our first chance to meet candidates so they need to show their personality. Is the personal statement important? Of course it is. There is a term that we use in application terms: value added. What can this student contribute to the university, the profession and society as a whole. That last point is incredibly important, particularly now as the government changes in the NHS have thrown physiotherapy to the forefront of outreach programmes to promote general health.*
>
> *Admissions tutor*

The personal statement

This is the most important part of your application, as this is where you convince the selectors that you are a serious and suitable candidate. Advice on writing your personal statement is given in the next chapter.

The reference

As well as your results and your personal statement, the selectors will take your reference into account. This is where your head, housemaster or housemistress, or head of Sixth Form writes about what an outstanding person you are – the life and soul of the school; how you are on target for three A grades at A level, and why you will become an outstanding physiotherapist. For him or her to say this, of course, it has to be true.

The referee is expected to be as honest as possible and to try to accurately assess your character and potential. You may believe that you have all of the qualities, both academic and personal, necessary in a physiotherapist, but unless you have demonstrated these to your teachers, they will be unable to support your application. Ideally, your efforts to impress them will have begun at the start of the Sixth Form (or before); you will have become involved in school activities, you will have been working hard at your studies, and you will be popular with students and teachers alike. However, it is never too late, and some people mature later than others, so if this does not sound like you, start to make efforts now to impress the people who will contribute to your reference.

As part of the reference, your referee will need to predict the grades that you are likely to achieve. If your predicted grades are lower than what is required for your chosen Physiotherapy courses, it is unlikely that you will be considered. Talk to your teachers and find out whether you are on target for the necessary grades. If not, you need to:

- work harder or more effectively – and make sure that your teachers notice that you are doing so, and/or;
- get some extra help either at school or outside, for instance, by taking an Easter revision course, and/or;
- delay submitting your UCAS application until you have your A level results. If you decide on this option, make sure that you use your gap year wisely (see below).

When to submit the UCAS application

The closing date for receipt of the application by UCAS for 2026 entry will be 14 January.

Late applications are accepted by UCAS, but the universities are not obliged to consider them. Because of the pressure on places, it is unlikely that late applications will be considered. Although you can submit your application any time between the beginning of September and the January deadline (remembering to get it to your referee at least two weeks before the deadline so that he or she has time to prepare the reference), most admissions tutors admit that the earlier the application is submitted, the better your chance of being called for an interview. Your best bet is to talk to the person who will deal with the application in the summer term of your first year of A levels and work on your personal statement and choice of universities over the summer holidays so that the application is ready to hand in at the start of the September term.

Deferred entry

Most admissions tutors are happy to consider students who take a gap year, and many encourage it. However, if you are considering this, you need to make sure that you are going to use the time constructively. A year spent watching daytime TV is not going to impress anybody, whereas independent travelling, charity or voluntary work either at home or abroad, work experience or a responsible job will all indicate that you have used the time to develop independence and maturity. Above all, make sure that whatever you do with the year involves regular contact with other people. It is a good idea to check with each individual institution that you are applying to whether they will accept a deferred application. Some advantages of a deferred year are that you can arrange to be overseas, either travelling or on a work or voluntary placement, without the worry of returning for college interviews. Also, it gives you another opportunity during this year to apply for other courses if your first application was unsuccessful.

You can either apply for deferred entry when you submit your UCAS application, in which case you need to outline your plans in your personal statement, or apply in the September following the publication of your A level results. If you expect to achieve your predicted grades and the feedback from your school or college is that you will be given a good reference, you should apply for deferred entry; but if you are advised by your referee that you are unlikely to be considered, you should give yourself more time to demonstrate to your referees that you have what it takes by waiting until you have your A level results.

What happens next?

You can follow the progress of your application using the UCAS online track system, which will show you when your form was sent to the universities and their responses.

The next correspondence you will receive, if you are lucky, is likely to be from the universities, asking you to attend an interview. Do not be alarmed if you do not hear anything soon after UCAS has sent you your statement of entry. Some universities interview on a first-come, first-served basis, while others wait until all applications are in before deciding whom to interview.

If you are unlucky, you will receive a message from UCAS telling you that you have been rejected by one or more of the universities. Do not despair; you may hear better news from another of the places that you applied to. Even if you get five rejections, the worst thing that you can do is give up and decide that it is no longer worth working hard. On the contrary, if this does happen, and you are not holding any offers, then you can still use UCAS Extra. This allows you to add another choice of university. If you are unsuccessful and did not achieve the grades required for the universities of your choice, then you will be automatically entered for Clearing on the UCAS website. The process of making Clearing applications is discussed in Chapter 8.

5 | Tweak it
The personal statement

Be interesting. That is the takeaway message from this chapter. Speak to any admissions tutor, and they will tell you that what they want is to read something that maintains their interest. Keep it factual and make it personal. What they are not looking for is a shopping list of your experiences. Look at everything from the point of view of, 'what has this gained me and how has it inspired me to do this course?'

The personal statement is your opportunity to demonstrate to the selectors that you have not only researched physiotherapy thoroughly but also have the right personal qualities to succeed as a physiotherapist. There are some universities that do not interview students, and therefore they need to see all the information that they are looking for in the personal statement. This chapter will guide you on what you should say and how you should say it.

For students applying to start their studies in 2026, personal statements are changing from one longer piece of text to three separate sections, each with a different question to help shape the focus for students' answers. Each of the three questions requires an answer that is at least 350 characters long (including spaces) and an overall maximum of 4,000 characters for the full personal statement.

Q1. Why do you want to study this course or subject?

A high proportion of UCAS applications contain the sentence: 'From an early age I have wanted to be a physiotherapist because it is the only career that combines my love of science with the chance to work with people.' Not only do admissions tutors get bored with reading this but it is also clearly untrue; if you think about it, there are many careers that combine science and people, including teaching, pharmacy, dentistry and nursing. However, the basic ideas behind this sentence may well apply to you.

You must use this section to demonstrate your knowledge and passion for physiotherapy. You could mention an incident that first got you interested – a visit to a physiotherapist, a conversation with a family friend or a lecture at school, for instance. You could write about your interest in human biology or about a biology project that you undertook when you were younger to illustrate your interest in science, and you could give examples of how you like to work with others. The important thing is to back up your initial interest in physiotherapy with your efforts to investigate the career.

Q2. How have your qualifications and studies helped you to prepare for this course or subject?

When writing this section of your personal statement for physiotherapy, focus on how your studies have prepared you for the course. Highlight relevant subjects, such as biology, which provides insight into anatomy, physiology and systems like the nervous and muscular systems, or chemistry, which enhances understanding of biochemistry and tissue repair. Mention how physical education or sports science has deepened your knowledge of exercise physiology and injury prevention, or how psychology has helped you understand motivation and mental health, crucial for patient care.

Include transferable skills developed through your studies, such as problem-solving, analytical thinking and effective communication. If you have undertaken independent research or projects related to health or biology, explain how these prepared you for university-level study. In this section, it is also important to highlight your proactive learning through workshops, lectures or online courses, showing your commitment to staying informed about developments in physiotherapy. Use specific examples to clearly connect your studies to your aspirations.

Q3. What else have you done to prepare outside of education, and why are these experiences useful?

An important aspect of this section is to describe your work experience. It is important to demonstrate that you gained something from the work experience and that it has given you an insight into the profession. You should indicate the length of time that you spent at each work placement, what treatments you observed and your impressions of physiotherapy.

You could comment on what aspects of physiotherapy attract you, what you found interesting or something that surprised you. Merely saying where you worked and what you saw is not enough; the selectors want to know what you learnt from the experience. Here is an example of a description of work experience that would not impress the selectors.

'I have spent six months volunteering at my local care home. Over this time I have seen various physiotherapy treatments, including ultrasounds, hydrotherapy and massages. I have also enjoyed learning how exercises can help the residents to maintain their mobility. Overall, it has been very interesting and informative.'

The next example would be much more convincing because it is clear that the student was interested in what was happening.

'During my six months volunteering at Oak Park care home, I was fortunate enough to shadow their resident physiotherapist. I watched a range of treatments, including ultrasound and exercise in the hydrotherapy pool. At Oak Park, they mainly used hydrotherapy as treatment for the residents with arthritis. It was especially beneficial for them as the warmth of the water allows their muscles to relax, allowing them to exercise as the pain in their joints was eased. As some of the residents are stroke victims, I also got to spend some time with a specialist neurological physiotherapist which was eye-opening. I learned that in these cases the physiotherapist has to physically assist the body in doing things it no longer has the ability to do itself, therefore these treatments are more hands-on and intense. I feel lucky to have had the chance to learn about a different branch of physiotherapy, as it was not an area I had come across before. Seeing first-hand the positive difference physiotherapy can make has only reaffirmed my goal to pursue a career as a physiotherapist.'

With luck, the selectors may pick up on this at the interview and ask questions about the methods that the physiotherapists used; the student could then bring in his or her knowledge of ultrasound (having investigated it following the work experience). This student would also gain extra credit with the admissions tutors for having arranged a lengthy work experience placement. Also, what admissions tutors look favourably on would be differing work experience placements, such as working with children or maybe disabled physiotherapy work. The greater the variety of work you have undertaken, the more attractive and interesting you are to the interviewer.

Extracurricular activities

In addition to work experience, you need the person reading your personal statement to know whether you have the qualities that they are looking for. They will expect to read about some of the following:

- participation in team events or general teamwork;
- involvement in school plays or concerts;
- positions of responsibility;
- work in the local community;
- Duke of Edinburgh Award;
- part-time or holiday jobs;
- charity work.

The selectors will be aware that some schools offer more in the way of activities and responsibilities than others, and they will make allowances for this. You do not have to have gone on a school expedition to India or to be head girl to be considered, but you need to be able to demonstrate that you have taken the best possible advantage of what is on offer. The selectors will be aware of the type of school or college that you have come from (there is a box on the back of the UCAS application that your referee fills in) and, consequently, of the opportunities that are open to you. What they are looking for is that you have grasped these opportunities. This section should be no longer than a paragraph long. Cover the key points you feel are important; you will have an opportunity to discuss these further at the interview.

TIP!

The person reading your UCAS application has to decide two things: whether you have the right personal qualities to become a successful physiotherapist, and whether you will cope with and contribute to university life.

Personal qualities

To be a successful physiotherapist, you need to be able to relate to other people; to survive and enjoy university, you need to be able to get on with a wide range of people too. Unlike school life, where many of the activities are organised and arranged by the teachers, almost all of the social activities at university are instigated and organised by the students. For this reason, the selectors are looking for people who have the enthusiasm and ability to motivate others and are prepared to give up their own time to arrange sporting, dramatic, musical or social activities.

It is also important to mention manual dexterity. Do you have any particular skills that show this, for example, playing a musical instrument, juggling or origami? Essentially, anything goes provided it shows your dexterous ability. After all, this is a career that involves you using your hands!

General tips

- Do not attempt to copy passages from other sources and incorporate them into your personal statement. UCAS uses anti-plagiarism software when checking statements; if you have used material from someone else (including the examples in this book), you will be caught out, and your application will be void.
- Do not be tempted to get someone else (a friend, teacher, parent or one of the many internet sites that offer 'help') to write your personal statement. It has to sound like you, which is why it is called a personal statement.
- Although you can apply for up to five institutions or courses, you write only one personal statement, and so it needs to be relevant to all of the courses you are applying for. You will not be able to write a convincing statement if you are applying to a variety of different courses.
- Print off a copy of your personal statement, so that you can remind yourself of all the wonderful things you said, should you be called for an interview!
- If you are applying for deferred entry, state your reasons for doing so and outline what you intend to do during your gap year. For example, you might be planning to find some relevant work experience in a private practice and then spend some time overseas volunteering with children.
- Do not be tempted to use overly formal or long-winded English.
- Read through a draft of your statement and ask yourself: 'Does it sound like me?' If not, rewrite it.

- Avoid phrases such as 'I was fortunate enough to be able to shadow a physiotherapist' when you really mean 'I shadowed a physiotherapist' or 'I arranged to shadow a physiotherapist'.
- Make sure you get someone else to read through it for you, perhaps your teacher or your parent/s. You can become so immersed in the personal statement that you don't see spelling mistakes or grammatical errors. A 'fresh set of eyes' is always best!

Using AI to support your personal statement

Artificial Intelligence (AI) refers to computer systems capable of performing tasks that usually require human intelligence. Tools like ChatGPT can generate human-like text and provide ideas for various tasks, including writing personal statements. However, using AI to assist in your personal statement requires careful consideration to ensure the final result remains authentic and personal.

Is using AI cheating?

Using AI tools like ChatGPT to generate and submit your entire personal statement as your own work can be considered dishonest and as cheating. UCAS requires applicants to declare that their personal statement is their original work and has not been copied or generated by AI. Statements that appear inauthentic or similar to others may be flagged by UCAS and universities or colleges will be notified. This could impact your chances of receiving an offer. The personal statement should showcase your unique skills, ambitions and experiences, qualities that AI cannot replicate.

How AI can help

While AI cannot replace your personal thoughts and voice, it can be a helpful tool if used appropriately. Here are some ways to use AI responsibly:

1. Idea Generation – AI can help you brainstorm relevant topics and experiences to include in your statement, providing a starting point for your writing process.
2. Structure – AI can suggest ways to organise your personal statement logically and effectively.
3. Proofreading – AI can aid in enhancing the clarity and readability of your statement by suggesting improvements in grammar, vocabulary and style.

Your personal statement, your voice

Universities and colleges value authenticity in personal statements. While AI tools are reshaping education and work, they cannot reflect your unique journey or convey your passion for your chosen course. Use AI tools to support your writing process, but ensure the final statement is a true representation of you. Writing your statement is a chance to confirm your aspirations and showcase your individuality, something no AI tool can replicate.

Sample personal statement 1

Why do you want to study this course or subject?

Physiotherapy is playing an ever more significant role in healthcare worldwide. Having studied biology, geography and food technology at A level, I have gained great insight into how a healthy, balanced lifestyle, through nutrition, exercise and health education, has led to increased longevity on a global scale. As healthcare costs rise and greater strain is put on clinics, surgeries and hospitals to provide treatment, I truly believe the future of medicine lies in preventative care, health promotion and rehabilitation.

My involvement in sports first sparked my interest in physiotherapy, but this broadened during an e-placement with the NHS Talent Academy, my first 'Introduction to Physiotherapy'. I was motivated by the chance to help not only athletes but patients across a wide range of profiles. This motivation grew stronger during my placement at Southampton General Hospital, where I witnessed the impact of physiotherapy in rehabilitation, such as helping an amputee walk on prosthetics shortly after surgery and providing care after heart attack complications. These experiences have inspired me to pursue a career in physiotherapy, where I can empower individuals to regain independence and improve their quality of life.

How have your qualifications and studies helped you to prepare for this course or subject?

Studying biology at A level has allowed me to learn more about human function, including how the nervous and circulatory systems work together to carry out key processes such as respiration and muscle contraction, which will be useful when studying physiotherapy. Through geography, I have seen how demography affects the life expectancy and healthcare demands of different countries, allowing me to discover a range of challenges faced within physiotherapy. Food technology has further enhanced my understanding of the importance of nutrition in maintaining a healthy lifestyle.

Together, these subjects have provided me with a strong foundation in understanding how lifestyle, education and preventative measures contribute to health and wellbeing, preparing me for physiotherapy's academic and practical demands.

What else have you done to prepare outside of education, and why are these experiences useful?

I undertook an e-placement with the NHS Talent Academy, which introduced me to the full breadth of knowledge physiotherapists require to tailor treatments for individual patients. My placement at Southampton General Hospital gave me insight into the immediate and long-term impact of physiotherapy in various settings, from cardiac recovery to amputee rehabilitation. Observing physiotherapy in animals, including horses and dogs, further developed my observational skills, as communication relied heavily on assessing non-verbal cues. Here, I also improved my communication and organisational skills by contacting patients, scheduling appointments and filing treatment notes.

Volunteering at Treloar's School for disabled children taught me how trust and communication are vital to physiotherapy, as I observed how a physiotherapist relied on a child's eye movements to assess their feelings and views on treatment. Similarly, at Riding for the Disabled and my local junior school, I enjoyed teaching children new skills, including reading, writing and horse riding. These experiences taught me patience and the importance of forming bonds, which are crucial in physiotherapy.

I seek to maintain a healthy and active lifestyle myself, regularly playing lacrosse and tennis at college and competing in horse riding at both individual and team levels. Earning my Gold Duke of Edinburgh Award has been a highlight, helping me develop commitment, leadership and teamwork skills, which are essential for physiotherapy.

Through all my experiences, I have gained a strong sense of purpose and motivation to enter a profession that provides independence and improves lives for those facing short-term or terminal illnesses.

Sample personal statement 2

Why do you want to study this course or subject?

I believe that there are two ways to consider disability: one is to focus on the lack of ability, and the other is to focus on the ability that remains. Growing up with disabled siblings taught me that a disability needn't define a person. Working within boundaries led to unique outcomes, and with every challenge disability brought, an opportunity arose. My sister who has Down's syndrome inspired me with her enthusiasm and positivity, while helping my deaf brother develop his confidence in speaking, and lip-reading gave me a deep appreciation for the potential to overcome challenges with the right guidance. These experiences instilled in me a compassionate and determined outlook that aligns with the core values of physiotherapy.

My personal experience with physiotherapy has been transformative. Diagnosed with a rare disorder that caused my knees to dislocate during flexion, I spent seven years training in the gym, developing innovative ways to strengthen my body and stabilise my joints. This journey not only gave me a completely normal life but also ignited my passion for fitness and compassion for those with physical limitations. Having received NHS physiotherapy for my condition, I witnessed the profound impact of tenacious and investigative care, which solidified my desire to pursue a career that improves lives and reduces the compromises society makes with its health.

How have your qualifications and studies helped you to prepare for this course or subject?

Studying biology at A level has been essential in building my understanding of physiotherapy. Exploring topics like the musculoskeletal and nervous systems has provided a solid foundation for comprehending how the body functions, moves and recovers. Practical experiments have further developed my analytical and problem-solving abilities. Through physical education, I gained valuable insights into exercise physiology and biomechanics, deepening my understanding of how physical activity influences recovery and performance. My coursework on injury prevention enhanced my interest in rehabilitation and offered me a clearer perspective on designing effective treatment strategies.

What else have you done to prepare outside of education, and why are these experiences useful?

During my time at Six Physio, a private network of physiotherapy clinics, I gained first-hand experience working with diverse clients. In my administrative support role for ten clinics in London, I learned to handle demanding situations with respect, dignity and kindness – qualities essential for physiotherapy. My interest in physiotherapy deepened as I explored the Oncology Department and researched the 2017 Macmillan report, Physical Activity and Cancer, which highlighted the benefits of physiotherapy in improving quality of life and physical outcomes for cancer patients. These experiences have provided me with valuable insight into how evidence-based practice can transform lives.

Travelling the world has also broadened my perspective, allowing me to witness poverty and primitive healthcare systems. This created a deep appreciation for the NHS and its role in society. My passion for physiotherapy was further strengthened by observing the physical and emotional benefits it provides, particularly in underserved areas like cancer rehabilitation. Learning that 60% of the 2 million people living with cancer in the UK have unmet physical needs has motivated me to contribute to addressing this demand within the NHS.

Whether it is facilitating simple rehab exercises for posture correction or designing post-cancer strength-conditioning programmes, my own journey through chronic pain and disability has given me the endurance and determination to empower patients to look beyond their limitations. Combining my personal insight with university knowledge, I hope to develop a career in physiotherapy that enables individuals to achieve independence and improved quality of life.

6| At full stretch
The interview

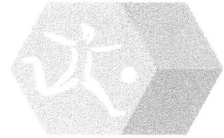

If the selectors like the picture that the UCAS application has painted of you, they may call you for an interview. The purpose of the interview is to allow them to see whether this picture is an accurate one and to investigate whether you have a genuine interest in physiotherapy. You must be aware of current events in the profession; this is discussed in Chapter 7. The interviewers will generally ask you three types of questions:

1. those designed to relax you so that they can assess your communication skills;
2. those designed to investigate your interest in and suitability for physiotherapy;
3. those designed to get a clearer picture of your personal qualities.

Sometimes the question will be no harder than 'Why this university?' However, that can catch many out, so make sure you have done even the basic research before your interview.

Questions to get you relaxed

'How was your journey here today?'

The interviewers are not really interested in the details of your travel. Do not be tempted to give them a minute-by-minute account of your bus journey ('and then we waited for six minutes at the road works on Corporation Street'), but also do not simply say 'OK'. Say something like, 'It was fine, thank you. The train journey took about two hours, which gave me the chance to catch up on some reading'. With a bit of luck, they will ask you what you read, which gives you the chance to talk about a book, newspaper, article or an item in *Frontline*, the magazine of the CSP.

'I am interested to know why you decided to apply to Grantchester'

Another variation on this might be: 'How did you narrow your choice down to five universities?' The panel will be looking for evidence of research and that your reasons are based on informed judgement.

Probably the best possible answer would start with 'I came to your open day', because you can then proceed to tell them why you like their university so much, what impressed you about the course and facilities, and how the atmosphere of the place would particularly suit you. Even if you are unable to attend open days, try to arrange a formal or informal visit before you are interviewed so that you can show that you are aware of the environment, both academic and physical, and that you like the place. If you know people who are at the university or on the course, so much the better.

You should also know about the course structure. In Chapter 2, there is an overview of the differences and similarities between courses, and the prospectus will give detailed information. Given the choice between a candidate who is not only going to make a good physiotherapist but clearly wants to come to their institution and another who may have the right qualities but does not seem to care whether he or she studies there or somewhere else, whom do you think the selectors will choose?

Answers to avoid include the following:

* 'Reputation' (unless you know in detail the areas for which the university is highly regarded).
* 'It's in London, and I don't want to move away from my friends.'
* 'You take a lot of retake students.'
* 'My dad says it is easy to get a place here.'

A good answer could be: 'I came to an open day last summer, which is why I have applied here. I enjoyed the day and was impressed by the facilities and by the comments of the students who showed us around because they seemed so enthusiastic about the course. Also, my cousin studied English at the university and I visited her and got to sample the atmosphere of the town.'

There are variations on this question. The interviewers may ask you what you know about the course or about the university. In all cases, this is your chance to show the interviewers that you are desperate to come to their university.

WARNING!

Do your homework by reading the prospectus and looking at the website. Although on the surface all Physiotherapy courses appear to cover broadly the same subjects, there are big differences in how the courses are delivered and in the opportunities for patient contact, and your interviewers will expect you to know about their course.

Questions about physiotherapy

'Why do you want to be a physiotherapist?'

This is the question that all interviewees expect. Given that the interviewers will be aware that you are expecting the question, they will also expect your answer to be planned carefully. If you look surprised and say something like 'Um . . . well . . . I haven't really thought about why', you can expect to be rejected. Other answers to avoid are: 'The money', 'I couldn't get into medicine', 'I want to help people' and 'I want to work for Arsenal'.

Many students are worried that they will sound insincere when they answer this question. The way to avoid this is to try to bring in reasons that are personal to you, for instance, an incident that started your interest (perhaps a visit to a physiotherapist) or an aspect of your work experience that particularly fascinated you. The important thing is to try to express clearly what interested you rather than to generalise your answers. Rather than say, 'Physiotherapy combines science, working with people and the chance to have control over your career', which says little about you, tell the interviewers about the way in which your interest progressed. Here is an example of a good answer.

'When I was involved with athletics for my club and taking part in events I also volunteered to help with the junior members of the team. From this came the opportunity to be involved with dealing with their injuries firsthand and assisting in their recovery, alongside the team physiotherapist. I always knew that I wanted to be involved with athletics even after my body has given up on me! Therefore, I saw becoming a physiotherapist as a great way to do this. I started taking an active commitment to learning more about physiotherapy by reading relevant materials and also volunteering at my local NHS physiotherapy ward.'

WARNING!

Do not learn this passage and repeat it at your interview. Ensure that your answer is not only personal to you but also honest.

With luck, the interviewers will pick up on something that you said about work experience and ask you more questions about this. Since 'Why do you want to be a physiotherapist?' is such an obvious question, interviewers often try to find out the information in different ways. Expect questions such as 'When did your interest in physiotherapy start?', 'What was it about your work experience that finally convinced you that physiotherapy was for you?' or 'I see that you spent two weeks with your physiotherapist. Was there anything that surprised you?'

Variations on this question could include 'Was there anything that particularly interested you?', 'Was there anything you found off-putting?' or simply 'Tell me about your work experience'. What these questions really mean is: 'Are you able to show us that you were interested in what was happening during your work experience?' To return to the original question, answering either 'Yes' or 'No' without explanation will not gain you many marks. Similarly, saying, 'Yes, I was surprised by the number of patients who seemed very scared', says nothing about your awareness of the physiotherapist's approach to his or her patients.

However, answering, 'Yes, I was surprised by the number of patients who seemed very scared. What struck me, however, was the way in which the physiotherapist dealt with each patient as an individual, sometimes being sympathetic, sometimes explaining things in great detail and sometimes using humour to relax them. For instance' shows that you were interested enough to be aware of more than the most obvious things.

Sentences that start with 'For example' and 'For instance' are particularly important, as they allow you to demonstrate your interest. In order to be able to give examples, you should keep a diary of things that you saw during your work experience so that you do not forget. You should read through this before your interview, as if you were revising for an examination.

'I see that you try to keep up to date with developments in physiotherapy. Can you tell me about something that you have read about recently?'

If you are interested in making physiotherapy your career, the selectors will expect you to be interested enough in the subject to want to read about it. Good sources of information are the CSP's website and others (addresses are given in Chapter 11), *Frontline* and the national newspapers. You should get into the habit of looking at a respected newspaper every day to see if there are any medical or physiotherapy-related stories.

Note that the question uses the word 'recently': recent does not mean an article you read two years ago – keep up to date. You could, for instance, say: 'There was a recent report that sportspeople risk injury from wearing air-filled training shoes. There was a survey of basketball players that showed that they were four times more likely to suffer ankle injuries if they were wearing trainers with soles that contained air pockets.'

'During your work experience, you had the chance to discuss physiotherapy with physiotherapists. What do you know about career opportunities and pay for physiotherapists?'

You must make sure that you do some research on career paths by asking questions about this when you meet physiotherapists.

Most physiotherapists work in the NHS, but there are many other options. In Chapter 1, we described many of the types of work undertaken by physiotherapists. Most physiotherapists end up specialising in one or more particular areas – in most cases as a result of an interest that grew during their training. The best answer to a question like this is to describe the career paths of physiotherapists you have met and worked with, as this will allow you to highlight your own work experience.

'What qualities should a physiotherapist possess?'

These have been discussed on page 47. However, do not simply list them. The question has not been asked because the interviewer is puzzled about what these qualities are; it has been asked to give you a chance to show:

- that you are aware of them, and
- that you possess them.

The best way to answer this is to use phrases such as 'During my work experience at the Grantchester Physiotherapy Clinic I was able to observe/talk to the physiotherapist, and I became aware that', or 'Communication is very important. For instance, when I was shadowing my physiotherapist, there was a patient who' Try always to relate these general questions to your own experiences.

'Physiotherapy requires high levels of physical fitness and manual dexterity. Do you possess these?'

Manual manipulation of a patient's limbs requires a fair degree of fitness and strength, and as a physiotherapist, you will need to be able to help to lift and lower patients. If you have trouble picking up a coffee cup without breathing heavily for the next 10 minutes, physiotherapy may not be the best career for you. The interviewers will need to be reassured that you are able to work in a physically demanding environment and also that you have the manual dexterity necessary to perform sometimes intricate tasks. Try to anticipate this question by preparing an answer that demonstrates that you have these qualities. Sport is always a good indicator of fitness and coordination, but you could also mention situations that you encountered during your work experience, demanding tasks that you perform as part of a weekend job, expeditions that you have been on at school as part of the Duke of Edinburgh's Award or a hobby such as DIY.

WARNING!

Do not lie about the example you describe. An admissions tutor I talked to recounted the story of an applicant who wrote in the UCAS application that he worked for a local Riding for the Disabled scheme. However, the previous interview had been with someone from the same town who had explained that there was no such scheme in the area, which is why she could not carry on doing this when she moved there. He was found out and rejected.

Questions to find out what sort of person you are

'What do you do to relax?'

Do not say 'watch TV' or 'go to the pub'. Mention something that involves working or communicating with others, for instance, sports or music. Use the question to demonstrate that you possess the qualities required in a physiotherapist. However, do not make your answer so insincere that the interviewers realise that you are trying to impress them. Saying, 'I relax most effectively when I go to the local physiotherapy clinic to shadow the physiotherapist', will not convince them.

'How do you cope with stress?'

Physiotherapy can be a stressful occupation. Physiotherapists have to deal with difficult people, those who are scared and those who react badly when in a physiotherapy ward. For many people, physiotherapy can be painful and distressing, and patients are not always cooperative or even aware of why they are receiving treatment. In these circumstances the physiotherapist cannot panic but must remain calm and rational. The interviewers will want to make a judgement as to whether you will be able to cope with the demands of the job.

Having been through them themselves, it is unlikely that they will regard school examinations as being particularly stressful. Hard work, yes, but not as stressful as training to be a physiotherapist or practising as a physiotherapist. What they are looking for are answers that demonstrate your calmness and composure when dealing with others. You could relate it to your work experience or your Saturday job. Dealing with a queue of angry and impatient customers demanding to know why their cheeseburgers are not ready can be difficult. Other areas that can provide evidence of stress management are school expeditions, public speaking or positions of responsibility at school or outside.

'I see that you enjoy reading. What is the most recent book that you have read?'

The question might be about the cinema or theatre, but the point of it is the same: to get you talking about something that interests you. Although it may sound obvious, if you have written in your UCAS application that you enjoy reading, make sure that you have actually read something recently. Admissions tutors will be able to tell you stories about interviewees who look at them with absolute amazement when they are asked about books, despite it being featured in the personal statement.

Answers such as 'Well . . . I haven't had much time recently, but . . . let me see . . . I read *Elle* last month, and . . . oh yes . . . I had to read *Jane Eyre* for my English GCSE' will do your chances no good at all. By all means put down that you like reading, but make sure that you have read an interesting novel in the period leading up to the interview, and be prepared to discuss it.

How to succeed in your interview

You should prepare for an interview as if you are preparing for an examination. This involves revision of your work experience diary so that you can recount details of your time with physiotherapists, revision of the newspaper, website and *Frontline* articles that you have saved, and revision of all of the things that you have mentioned on your personal statement.

> *Although I was nervous before my interview, I think I was prepared enough to answer all the questions well. I had been advised by a teacher to take my time and think about the question, rather than rush in to an answer, which was good advice. I also had some questions prepared for the end of the interview. I asked about dropout rates and work placements, which I believe showed the interviewer that I was both prepared and serious about the course.*
> *Simon, University of Sussex*

When you are preparing for your A levels, you sit a mock examination so that the real thing does not come as a total surprise; when you are preparing for an interview, have a mock interview so that you can get some feedback on your answers. Your school may be able to help you. If not, independent sixth-form colleges usually provide a mock interview service. Friends of your parents may also be able to help. If possible, video your mock interview so that you are aware of the way you come across in an interview situation. There is a list of practice interview questions overleaf.

Mock interview questions

Questions about you (general)
- Why do you want to be a physiotherapist?
- Why does physiotherapy interest you more than medicine/nursing/radiography?
- What are the ideal qualities that a physiotherapist should possess, and do you think you possess those qualities?
- Give me an example of how you cope with stress.
- What have you done to demonstrate your commitment to the community?
- What would you contribute to this university?
- What are your best/worst qualities?
- What was the last novel you read? What did you think of it?
- What was the last play/film you saw? What did you think of it?
- What do you do to relax?
- What is your favourite A level subject?
- What grades do you expect to gain in your A levels?
- What branch of physiotherapy interests you the most and why?
- Why are you taking a gap year?

Questions related to your research into physiotherapy/the university and relevant work experience (example/anecdotal)
- What have you done to investigate physiotherapy?
- Why did you apply to this university?
- Did you come to our open day?
- During your work experience, did anything surprise or shock you?
- Was the physiotherapist you shadowed good at communicating with his/her patients?
- Have you read any articles about physiotherapy recently?
- Why are communication skills important for physiotherapists?
- What have you done that demonstrates your communication skills?
- What have you done that demonstrates your leadership skills?
- What have you done that demonstrates your ability to cope in a stressful situation?
- How did you organise your work experience?
- How does teamwork apply to the role of a physiotherapist?

Questions about physiotherapy (academic)
- Tell me about preventative physiotherapy.
- What is occupational therapy?
- What is repetitive strain injury?
- What is cystic fibrosis/a stroke/arthritis?
- What is hydrotherapy?

- What is ultrasound, and how is it used?
- Is exercise always good for you?
- How much do NHS physiotherapists earn?
- What advances can we expect in physiotherapy technology/ treatment in the future?
- What precautions need to be taken with patients who are HIV positive?
- What is the role of a physiotherapist in a hospital?
- Why is a knowledge of physics helpful in physiotherapy?
- What are the particular difficulties that animal physiotherapists encounter?

MMIs

There is a growing use of Multiple Mini Interviews (MMIs) now at the application stage. For example, University of Nottingham interviews are conducted online using the web-based SAMMI-Select© software. This is a MMI online platform, where you will be asked a range of pre-recorded questions.

If you are going to attend an MMI, then it is a good idea to ask multiple members of staff at your school to ask you different questions and get you to think on your feet.

Sample MMI questions
Station #1:

PROMPT (Read and consider for 2 minutes):

A friend tells you that her dad has been battling alcoholism for years, and it has put a strain on the family. They are thinking they will have to leave their studies and go home to help out in the family as it is all too much right now. How do you counsel your friend?

RESPOND: (Speak max. 8 minutes)

Station #2:

PROMPT (Read and consider for 2 minutes):

What do you think are the major sorts of problems facing a person with a long-term health problem, such as arthritis?

RESPOND: (Speak max. 8 minutes)

Station #3:

PROMPT (Read and consider for 2 minutes):

Imagine you are on a committee able to recommend only one of two new treatments to be made available through the NHS. The treatments are an artificial heart for babies born with heart defects or a permanent replacement hip for people with severe arthritis. Both treatments are permanent, i.e. never need repeating, and are of equal cost. On what grounds would you make your arguments?

RESPOND: (Speak max. 8 minutes)

Station #4:

PROMPT (Read and consider for 2 minutes):

Can you think of something you'd like to invent?

RESPOND: (Speak max. 8 minutes)

Station #5:

PROMPT (Read and consider for 2 minutes):

Give us an example of something about which you used to hold strong opinions but have had to change your mind. What made you change? What do you think now?

RESPOND: (Speak max. 8 minutes)

Appearance and body language

Appearance and body language are important. The impression you create can be very influential. Remember that if the interviewers cannot picture you as a physiotherapist in future years, they are unlikely to offer you a place.

Body language
- Maintain eye contact with the interviewers.
- Direct most of what you are saying to the person who asked you the question, but occasionally look around at the others on the panel.
- Sit up straight, but adopt a position that you feel comfortable in.
- Do not wave your hands around too much, but do not keep them gripped together to stop them from moving. Fold them across your lap, or rest them on the arms of the chair.

Speech
- Talk slowly and clearly.
- Do not use slang.
- Avoid saying 'erm', 'you know' or 'sort of'.
- Say 'hello' at the start of the interview, and 'thank you' and 'goodbye' at the end.

Dress and appearance
- Wear clothes that show you have made an effort for the interview.
- You do not have to wear a business suit, but a jacket and tie or a skirt and shirt/blouse are appropriate.
- Make sure that you are clean and tidy.

- If appropriate, shave before the interview (but avoid overpowering aftershave).
- Clean your nails and shoes.
- Wash your hair.
- Avoid (visible) piercings, earrings, jeans and trainers.

Online interviews

Over recent years, universities have been using online interviews, and these require thoughtful preparation to ensure your appearance and body language create a professional and confident impression, even through a screen. The interviewers should be able to picture you as a future physiotherapist, demonstrating professionalism, empathy and communication skills.

- Look directly at the camera when speaking to simulate eye contact, rather than at the screen or your own image.
- Avoid slouching or leaning too close to the camera.
- Use natural hand gestures when appropriate, but keep them within the frame of the camera.
- Speak slowly and clearly to ensure you are easily understood through the microphone.
- Wear formal or semi-formal attire, such as a shirt/blouse and jacket. Avoid overly casual clothing, even if only your upper body is visible.
- Use a neutral or tidy background to keep the focus on you. If possible, sit in front of a plain wall or use a virtual background if it is appropriate and professional.
- Ensure your face is well-lit, ideally by natural light or a soft lamp positioned in front of you. Avoid strong backlighting.
- Position your camera at eye level so you appear natural and engaged.
- Test your microphone beforehand to ensure clear sound quality and avoid background noise.

At the end of the interview

You may be given the opportunity to ask a question at the end of the interview. Bear in mind that the interviews are carefully timed, and that your attempts to impress the panel with 'clever' questions may do quite the opposite. The golden rule is: ask a question only if you are genuinely interested in the answer (which, of course, you were unable to find during your careful reading of the prospectus).

Questions to avoid
- 'What is the structure of the first year of the course?'
- 'Will I be able to live in a hall of residence?'
- 'When will I first have contact with patients?'

As well as being boring questions, the answers to these will be available in the prospectus. You have obviously not done any serious research.

Questions you could ask

- 'Are my A levels enough of a foundation before starting this course or could you recommend something else I should review before starting?' Proactive.
- 'Do you think I should try to get more work experience before the start of the course?' Again, an indication of your keenness.
- 'Earlier, I couldn't answer the question you asked me on ultrasound. What is the answer?' Something that you genuinely might want to know.
- 'How soon will you let me know if I have been successful or not?' Something you really want to know.

REMEMBER!

If in doubt, do not ask a question. End by saying, 'All of my questions have been answered by the prospectus and the students who showed me around the university. Thank you very much for an interesting day.' Smile, shake hands (if appropriate – if you are being interviewed by a panel of five, who are all sitting at the other end of a long table, then do not!), and say goodbye.

Structuring the interview

The selectors will have a set of questions that they may ask, designed to assess your suitability and commitment. If you answer 'Yes' or 'No' to most questions, or reply only in monosyllables, they will fire more and more questions at you. If, however, your answers are longer and also contain statements that interest them, they are more likely to pick up on these, and you are, effectively, directing the interview. If you are asked questions that you have prepared for, there will be less time for the interviewers to ask you questions that might be more difficult to answer.

For example, at the end of your answer to a question about work experience, you might say, 'and the physiotherapist was able to explain the effect of new technology on physiotherapy.' The interviewer may then say, 'I see. Can you tell me about how technology is changing physiotherapy?' You can then embark on an answer about ultrasound, for instance. At the end of your explanation, you could finish with: 'of course, ultrasound treatment is often used in conjunction with infrared radiation treatment.' You might then be asked about situations where this might happen, and so on.

Of course, this does not always work, but you would be very unlucky not to have at least one of these 'signposts' followed that you placed in front of the interviewers.

How you are selected

During the interview, the panel will be assessing you in various categories. Whether or not the interview appears to be structured, the interviewers will be following careful guidelines so that they can compare candidates from different interview sessions. Some panels adopt a conversational style, whereas others are more formal. The scoring system will vary from place to place, but, in general, you will be assessed in the following categories:

- reason for your choice of university;
- academic ability;
- motivation for physiotherapy;
- awareness of physiotherapy issues;
- personal qualities;
- communication skills.

You are likely to be scored in each category, and the university will have a minimum mark that you will have to gain if you are to be made an offer. If you are below this score but close to it, you may be put on an official or unofficial waiting list. If this happens, you may be considered in August, should there be places available.

If you are offered a place, you will receive a notification on UCAS Hub from the university telling you what you need to achieve in your A levels. This is called a conditional offer. Post-A level students who have achieved the necessary grades will be given unconditional offers. If you are unlucky, all you will get is an email from UCAS saying that you have been rejected. If this happens, it is not necessarily the end of the road that leads you to a career in physiotherapy.

If you are rejected by all of your choices, you can enter the UCAS Extra scheme, which allows you to contact other universities. If you still are without a place when the A level results are released in August, you will be eligible to apply for vacant places through Clearing.

When UCAS has received replies from all of your choices, it will send you a Statement of Offers. You will then have about a month to make up your mind about where you want to go. If you have only one offer, you will have little choice but to accept it. If you have more than one, you will have to accept one as your firm choice and another (usually a lower offer) as your insurance choice. If the place where you really want to study makes a lower offer than one of your other choices, do not be tempted to choose the lower offer as your insurance choice, since you will be obliged to go to the university that you have put as your firm choice if you achieve the grades. Even if you narrowly miss the grade, you may still be accepted by your first choice. If you decide that you do not want to go there, once the results are issued, you will have to withdraw from the UCAS system for that year.

It's so important that prospective students understand what physiotherapists do. They have to comprehend the depth of the job. Prospective students need to show compassion and motivation. When people are in pain it's not easy to get them moving. You have to show empathy rather than sympathy.

Admissions Tutor

7 | Do you know your gluteus maximus from your articulatio cubiti?
Current issues

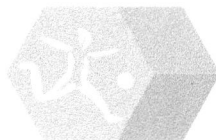

This chapter explains the most relevant current issues in physiotherapy. This should be used as a reference point for your interview but not as your only source of information. You should make sure that you read newspapers and journals (such as *Frontline*) to get ideas on other current issues and not just rely on those listed here. Your success at the interview will depend on your ability to converse fluently on up-to-date topics. You do not have to be an expert in your field – that is what the interviewers are – but you do need to have tried to understand the profession that you wish to follow. If that comes as a surprise, this is not the right career for you!

The NHS Long-Term Plan

With the NHS turning 70 years old in 2019, the NHS Long-Term Plan, first published in January 2019, aimed to ensure its future success. The plan sets out a range of aims to make sure everyone gets the best start in life, to deliver world-class care for major health problems and to support people into their older years. There was to be improved funding of 3.4% over the following five years, compared to 2.2% over the previous five years. The plan was put into effect after consulting patients' groups, professional bodies and frontline NHS leaders.

In relation to physiotherapy, the plan saw the physiotherapy workforce as key to successfully delivering the changes, with prevention and rehabilitation at the forefront. Furthermore, there is support for increasing the number of personnel to deal with primary and community care, along with the increase of funding.

This launch, by NHS England's Simon Stevens, has been seen as a major breakthrough for physiotherapy and the treatment of patients. A promise to create many more first contact physiotherapist roles and wider access to rehabilitation across a range of conditions sees a number of positive references to the profession.

Professor Karen Middleton, chief executive of the CSP, said:

> 'It marks the clear shift towards providing services in the community that we have long called for, and places an emphasis on prevention.
>
> 'It explicitly sets out the integral role physiotherapy staff, including first contact physiotherapists, will make in delivering this transformation.
>
> 'Crucially, it also sets out targets on rehabilitation across a number of conditions, which will serve to focus minds when designing and commissioning services.
>
> 'We will go through the detail in the coming days and it is already obvious that there remain unanswered questions about workforce and social care funding, among other issues. These must be addressed if we are to achieve the success the plan aspires to.
>
> 'But as a blueprint for how the NHS should proceed with physiotherapy playing a crucial role, there is a lot to like in this plan.'
>
> Information taken from the CSP (www.csp.org.uk), with kind permission from the CSP.

The points listed below highlight the key implications for physiotherapy as a result of the NHS England Long-Term Plan.

Overall

- Prevention and rehabilitation are key themes throughout the plan.
- The physiotherapy workforce is identified as essential to successfully delivering the plan.
- There is support for expanding the physiotherapy workforce in primary and community care.
- There is a commitment to increasing the funding of both primary and community services as a proportion of the overall health budget.
- Digital infrastructure will be deployed to improve data collection, access to services, personal health records and to support self-care.
- There is a commitment to invest in physiotherapy workforce development. However, specific commitments on CPD and career development are still focused on nurses and doctors.
- There is no mention at all of the unregistered physio/Allied Health Professions (AHP) workforce.

Primary care

- The first contact physio (FCP) model will be endorsed as part of a new vision for integrated primary and community services. It will be implemented beyond the existing pilots.
- FCPs will be part of the 'GP Forward View' workforce targets for the first time.
- Physiotherapists will be part of the primary care workforce in rapid response teams.
- Digital technology will enable GP appointments to be bookable via NHS 111.
- Primary care networks will have a role in the early diagnosis of Chronic Obstructive Pulmonary Disease (a similar approach to the frailty index in General Practice).

Community rehabilitation

- Community rehabilitation is highlighted as an area for significant development.
- There is a proposal for integrated community hubs, with physiotherapy as part of multidisciplinary teams.
- There is a specific commitment to expand pulmonary, cardio and stroke rehabilitation.
- Needs assessments for stroke and cancer patients will include rehabilitation after discharge.

Information taken from the CSP (www.csp.org.uk),
with kind permission from the CSP.

The NHS England Long-Term Plan contains many encouraging ideas and directives for all those involved in and around physiotherapy. Patients will be able to book convenient appointments directly with physios and other expert health professionals at a local practice, without the need to wait for a referral or travel to a specialist clinic.

Professor Stephen Powis, NHS National Medical Director, said: 'More physios based in community GP surgeries means people have more choice and can get the treatment they need without waiting weeks to make what can be a long journey to hospital for a short appointment, and is a great example of how the NHS Long-Term Plan will increasingly deliver more care options closer to home over the coming years.'

Concussion

Despite being in the spotlight for a few years already, the 2022 Football World Cup in Qatar once again drew attention to how concussion appears to be overlooked in elite football after Iran's goalkeeper was allowed to play on despite suffering a head injury that took ten minutes to treat. Physiotherapists can continue to play a key role in educating sportsmen and women about concussion.

Clinical update: Concussion

According to a report in the CSP's *Frontline* magazine, minor head trauma isn't just a sports injury:

> 'Physios in all specialisms can help to spot undiagnosed concussion that needs treatment.

> 'Concussion is a minor traumatic brain injury caused by a blow to the head or violent head movement, such as in a traffic collision. Although there is often no outward damage, and the patient usually stays conscious, the jolt may briefly disrupt electrical activity in the brain.

> 'It's more common among sports players, young men, older people and those who are homeless or have mental health problems. Children and teenagers take longer to recover and are more likely to suffer long-term damage. Having concussion more than once increases the risk of long-term damage.

> 'Among sports players, evidence suggests that women are more likely to have concussion, and that the risk may be related to the menstrual cycle, with experts noting that sportswomen often recover slower from concussion than sportsmen.

> 'Anyone suffering a head injury should be monitored over several days as bleeding inside the skull is not immediately obvious.

> 'In sport, there are new laws around head injuries. Any head injury should be treated as serious and the player be immediately removed from the field of play and not allowed to return during the match. They should then be properly medically assessed. There should be a minimum period of one week's rest and then the Graduated Return To Play programme is applied, once the symptoms have stopped. This is a minimum of one week and they need to be carefully monitored by medical staff and physiotherapists.'

> *Information taken from the CSP (www.csp.org.uk), with kind permission from the CSP.*

The role of a physiotherapist

All physiotherapists in any field may find themselves in the situation of saving a life. Any bump on the head could cause minor brain trauma, and this could lead to bigger problems in the future. Physiotherapists can pick up on signs or indicators that a patient might be suffering more than they let on, or even perhaps more than they know. A good example in physiotherapy is that of vestibular rehabilitation. This is used in the treatment of a loss of balance, but if a concussion is involved, the patient may be suffering from other after-effects that require looking at and possible treatment.

Symptoms to look out for are drowsiness, dizziness, nausea, headache or pressure in the head, loss of memory, difficulty in understanding or communicating and sensitivity to light or noise. If they are encountering severe neck pain, deteriorating consciousness, increasing confusion or irritability, severe headache, repeated vomiting, unusual behaviour, convulsions, problems with seeing or hearing or weakness or tingling in arms or legs, then you should seek immediate medical attention.

The approach to managing concussions more safely is gaining traction across various sports, with players now being routinely removed from play following a suspected concussion. Organisations such as the Football Association (FA) and England Rugby have introduced strict guidelines in recent years, allowing physiotherapists to overrule Premier League managers seeking to return players to the field prematurely.

Technology in physiotherapy

Enter the words 'physiotherapy' and 'news' into an internet search engine, and most of the links that you get are to news stories about new forms of treatment. Although the basic techniques used in physiotherapy have been around for a long time – physical manipulation, repetition of exercises and other forms of manual therapy – technology plays an increasingly important role.

Probably the most widely used application of technology within physiotherapy is ultrasound. Ultrasound treatment utilises high-frequency (up to 3MHz – too high for the human ear to hear) sound waves. Ultrasound is used extensively in medicine for diagnosis, either to form images in order to see what is happening inside the body (for instance, scans that show a foetus inside the womb) or to measure blood flow.

Whenever ultrasound waves pass from one tissue to another, a small percentage of the beam is reflected back, and these reflected sound waves are used to create a picture or to measure the speed at which blood is flowing (using something called the Doppler effect). Ultrasound can also be used therapeutically; that is, for treatment. It has been used to accelerate tissue repair and to relieve pain since the 1950s. It is used to treat a variety of conditions, such as sports injuries, sprains, tendonitis, arthritis and ulcers, and to relieve the pain associated with, for instance, phantom limbs in amputees. The sound waves penetrate deep into the body, and, although the biological effects are not completely understood, it is likely that the vibration caused by the sound waves produces a combination of heating (thermal effects) and stimulation of tissue and blood vessels (mechanical effects). Ultrasound is usually given at the end of a course of treatment, following other forms of manual therapy.

Ultrasound equipment is relatively cheap to buy (less than £2,000 for an ultrasound machine) and is easy to use. The drawbacks of the extensive use of ultrasound in physiotherapy are that there is little conclusive clinical evidence that it is effective and that there is a possible risk of tissue damage if the power settings on individual machines are not calibrated accurately.

Another treatment that utilises sound waves, extracorporeal shockwave therapy (ESWT), has been introduced into physiotherapy clinics. ESWT was brought to a wider audience in 2004 when Sachin Tendulkar, the Indian cricketer, received shockwave therapy to treat tennis elbow that had failed to respond to conventional physiotherapy. Developed from the devices that generate pulses of sound waves to destroy kidney stones, ESWT devices produce pulses of high-pressure sound that travel through the skin. Soft tissue and bone that are subjected to these pulses of high-pressure energy heal back stronger. Tennis elbow results from calcification of a tendon and is usually treated with mechanical exercise or steroid injection (which risks weakening the tendon still further), but new treatments are also being developed.

There are instances of robots being used in physiotherapy. This does not mean that next time you require physiotherapy, you will be treated by R2-D2, Bender or Kryton. The effective rehabilitation of patients with cerebral palsy, or following a stroke or other brain injuries, requires repetitive movement exercises and controllable resistance to motion. In one such treatment, the patient is coupled to a robot joystick that guides him or her through a series of movements. The robot can be programmed to vary the scope of the movement, to increase or decrease the resistance, or to help the patient to complete the movements. To increase interest levels for the patient, the movements can be integrated into a 'game' on a screen in front of the patient. In this way, tens of thousands of therapeutic movements can be completed over the course of a few weeks – far more than the physiotherapist could manage and more than the patient is likely to be able to accomplish alone.

One of the biggest and most comprehensive advances in physiotherapy is The Performance Matrix (TPM). This is a collection of analytical software that identifies the weak points and high-risk areas of your movement, such as your back or joints. TPM involves performing roughly 15 movement tests to identify these points, the results of which are calculated immediately. TPM is used to aid rehabilitation and recovery, as well as injury prevention. For this reason, it has proven popular not just with people who have sustained an injury but also with professional athletes looking to maximise their performance.

Though still a relatively young technology, virtual reality (VR) is providing a lot of exciting opportunities for all sorts of different medical professionals. One of the biggest advantages of this is the immersiveness of VR, which enables people in remote areas to exercise as if they were in a class full of people. It also helps monitor their movements and keep them on the right track. Additionally, VR can be used to make the exercises much more fun and even something people enjoy, making patients more likely to stick with their regimen. You can expect to see VR become commonplace in the next few years.

Another technological advance for physiotherapy is the creation of apps that are designed to help people address their physiotherapy issues independently. For example, there is one app that allows you to locate over 100 trigger points in over 70 muscles, and another that helps you to understand prevention of future medical needs; one that corrects spinal posture; and another that measures range of motion. In this modern age, millions of people are wearing fitness tracker watches and wristbands to measure their steps, heart rate and general levels of activity. This information can be used to calculate and track a range of other things, such as how many calories you've burned.

AI is increasingly being integrated into physiotherapy to enhance patient care and improve outcomes. AI applications include motion analysis, where algorithms assess patients' movements to identify abnormalities, and virtual physiotherapy platforms that use AI to tailor exercise plans. A significant milestone in the UK is the trial of the country's first AI-powered physiotherapy clinic, launched by NHS Lothian in July 2024. This clinic leverages AI to support musculoskeletal care by analysing patient data and providing real-time feedback on rehabilitation exercises. Running as a pilot programme, the initiative aims to reduce waiting times and improve accessibility while maintaining high-quality care. If successful, this trial could pave the way for wider adoption of AI in physiotherapy services across the NHS, blending human expertise with cutting-edge technology.

Mental health

Research has been undertaken that demonstrates that around one in five people with osteoarthritis has suffered from depression or anxiety at one time or another. Also, a third of people who have suffered a stroke have endured a depressive episode. If physiotherapists fail to recognise symptoms while working with recovering patients, then the results could be fatal.

Valuing the physical health of people with mental health issues is essential to patient rehabilitation and continuing progress. Mental health challenges can significantly impact physiotherapy, as they may slow recovery, hinder adherence to treatment plans, and heighten pain sensitivity, creating distinct difficulties in care. Furthermore, the nature of the profession – handling emotionally demanding cases, managing heavy workloads and maintaining compassionate communication – can lead to increased stress and burnout among physiotherapists.

As healthcare shifts towards a more holistic approach, physiotherapists are increasingly required to address mental health factors alongside physical rehabilitation, emphasising the importance of mental health awareness and support within the field. Patients undertaking around 120 minutes a week of physical activity are around 30% less likely to develop depression or anxiety in the future.

An ageing population

In 2022, there were around 12.7 million people aged 65 or over in the UK, making up 19% of the population. According to the ONS's population projections, by 2072 this could rise to 22.1 million people, or 27% of the population. By contrast, 50 years ago in 1972 there were around 7.5 million people aged 65 or over, or 13% of the population.

Information taken from the House of Commons Library website (www.commonslibrary.parliament.uk/the-uks-changing-population/)

Contains Parliamentary information licensed under the Open Parliament Licence v3.0.

At present, there is a strain on physiotherapy services, which have to deal with the effects of ageing and mobility among the elderly. Physiotherapy services therefore need to focus on facilitating independence among the elderly so that they are not dependent on the health services or care facilities to cope with normal life. Physiotherapy should also enable those still of working age to continue working, thus reducing the need for early retirement. A factsheet on musculoskeletal disorders (MSDs) published by the CSP highlights that MSDs are the most common physiotherapy problem treated among the workforce and are therefore a priority to be addressed in order to prevent further problems down the line.

Prescribing more activity for older people is part of a more proactive approach by physiotherapists to prevent a loss of mobility and independence.

A 2015 article in the *Guardian* newspaper states that 'Starting an exercise regime in your 70s or 80s may sound unusual. But for a growing number of older people it could help them hold on to their independence for longer, and reduce the pressure on families, carers and the health and social care system.' The article goes on to explain in more detail how this can be achieved. '"There is a lot of evidence that physical activity and exercise are valuable however old you are, and that frail, older people gain the most benefit," says Louise McGregor, vice-chair of the Agile professional network for physiotherapists working with older people. "You are really never too old. We now have a lot more people who live into their 100s and they can still benefit from the right type of exercise."'

Another area where physiotherapy could have a lasting benefit is with people with dementia. Physiotherapists can have a key role in assessing a patient's needs and giving high-quality care. Louise McGregor says that creative, adaptable strategies are important for such patients, as while an elderly person with dementia would benefit from a physiotherapy or exercise programme, they may well forget to follow it.

Obesity

Obesity is one of the biggest health challenges that we face in this country. It is an issue that the government is now actively trying to combat, as 26.2% of adults in the UK are currently obese, and a further 37.8% are overweight. Statistics from the BMJ report indicated that if the trend continues, then by 2030, 35% of adults are expected to be obese, the highest in Europe. The annual cost to the NHS is estimated to be £6.5 billion, and the social annual cost (i.e. cost to society) in the UK is around £58 billion. These sums have jumped significantly in recent years, partly due to the Covid-19 pandemic.

As we have already discussed, prevention is just as important as cure. In August 2016 a government 'childhood obesity strategy' was published highlighting the dangers of high sugar intake. In 2018, sugar levies on soft drinks were introduced, as well as guidance on calorie-reduction programmes. This was preceded by schemes such as the healthy-eating Change4Life movement, nowadays named Healthier Families. The CSP recommends that an adult should exercise five times a week at moderate intensity for roughly 30 minutes. If that is not physically possible, that is, you have time constraints that do not allow a concentrated period of exercise, then manage your time effectively and split the 30 minutes into shorter sessions at different intervals throughout the day. It may sound obvious, but this will have a positive effect on your health if continued over a long period of time.

The campaign is designed to show people that increased levels of physical activity can prevent, or help to control, more than 20 medical conditions, most notably obesity, osteoarthritis, heart disease, type 2 diabetes and other conditions affecting wellbeing such as depression. If nothing else, the release of endorphins through increased levels of activity will have a positive effect on productivity and output during a working day. It is a complete endorsement of the adage 'healthy body, healthy mind'.

Childhood obesity

Childhood obesity and excess weight are significant health issues for children and their families, as there can be serious implications for a child's physical and mental health, which can continue into adulthood. The number of children with an unhealthy and potentially dangerous weight is a national public health concern. Healthcare professionals play an important role in supporting families to take action. Working alongside physiotherapists and other public health teams, they can also influence the population as a whole by delivering systemic approaches to tackle excess weight and help reduce drivers of excess calorie intake and sedentary lifestyles.

The statistics are compelling, and the pandemic-related lockdowns in 2020 and 2021 worsened further young people's participation in physical activity. Sport England found that fewer than half now participate in at least 60 minutes of physical activity per day, while almost half do not even achieve 30 minutes. A 2022 study by Swansea University also found children in Wales to be among the least active in the world. The website www.kidshealth.org has great recommendations on how children can improve their health with simple and effective ideas.

A government report on childhood obesity stated that: 'Low levels of physical activity, and increased sedentary behaviours among children and young people, exacerbate the problems of poor diet and nutrition. Boys are more likely than girls to meet the recommended levels, as are children from the most affluent families when compared with the least affluent families.'

Parkinson's disease

Parkinson's is a progressive neurological condition characterised by motor and non-motor problems. The main changes arise from brain dysfunction through reduced production of chemical messengers, particularly the neurotransmitter dopamine.

Drug therapy and deep brain stimulation can provide partial relief of symptoms, but many people require additional support from allied health interventions, including physiotherapy, which was rated as a top priority by respondents to the membership survey conducted by the charity Parkinson's UK.

Physiotherapy involvement is supported by a growing evidence base of high-quality research, which is informing best practice guidelines. Short-term patient benefits in a range of physical and quality-of-life measures have been identified through systematic reviews.

Physiotherapy assessment and management focuses on improving physical capacity and quality of movement in daily life through walking and transfer training, balance and falls education, and practice of manual activities (e.g. reaching and grasping). Other issues, for example, pain, wellbeing, respiratory function and support networks, may need attention.

The two main areas of Parkinson's-specific physiotherapy intervention relate to exercise and movement strategy training. During the earlier stages, physiotherapists emphasise education and self-management, encouraging the use of leisure and third-sector programmes that promote general fitness and inclusion in community activity. Physiotherapy-specific exercise can offset the effects of Parkinson's to minimise deterioration in strength, endurance, flexibility and balance.

As the condition progresses, physiotherapists teach and apply movement strategies to overcome difficulty in generating automatic movement and thought, including developing strategies to compensate for loss of function, using external (auditory, tactile, visual and sensory) or internal (mental rehearsal and visualisation) cues, dual-task training, self-instruction and improving attention span.

Physiotherapy is essential in the multidisciplinary management of people with Parkinson's. Advice and education offered in the early stages maintain general fitness, minimise deterioration and promote self-management. In the later stages, physiotherapy can improve gait, balance, transfers and manual activities and reduce the falls risk.

Information taken from the CSP (www.csp.org.uk),
with kind permission from the CSP.

Repetitive strain injury

Repetitive strain injury (RSI) is an increasingly common complaint among computer users. As the name suggests, the condition is caused by repetition of certain movements, usually associated with computer keyboard use. However, RSI is not confined to computer users and has been diagnosed in many people whose jobs involve manual labour or machine operation. Prevalence has been especially noted within the armed forces and among construction, textile processing and other processing workers. The condition can also occur when the person's posture is inappropriate to the task that he or she is undertaking. It is recognised as one of the most common workplace injuries, with a recent survey reporting that 500,000 UK workers have reported an RSI, resulting in a total loss of 5.4 million working days a year.

RSI manifests itself as pain, mostly when the task that caused it is being carried out, but often at other times as well. It usually affects the neck, shoulders, elbows, wrists or hands. RSI is also known by other names, including WRMSD (work-related musculoskeletal disorder), WRULD (work-related upper limb disorder), CTD (cumulative trauma disorder) and OOS (occupational overuse syndrome). The term RSI actually encompasses a number of different conditions, most commonly carpal tunnel syndrome. 'Carpal' comes from the Greek word *karpos*, which means wrist. The joint in the wrist is surrounded by fibrous tissue, and there is a small gap between this tissue and the bone, through which a nerve (the median nerve) passes. The nerve then splits to serve the fingers and thumb. Repetitive movement of the wrist can cause swelling of the tissue in the wrist, putting pressure on the median nerve. Symptoms include numbness and tingling in the fingers and thumb, followed by pain. The condition can usually be cured by a combination of physiotherapy and rest.

Not everyone believes that RSI actually exists. Carpal tunnel syndrome certainly does, and it can be caused by obesity, arthritis, diabetes and pregnancy, but some people are sceptical as to whether repetitive movement is a cause. A report in the *British Medical Journal* on research done at Manchester University cast some doubts on RSI. The research indicated that the majority of those who suffered from arm or wrist pain (105 people in a survey involving 1,200 volunteers) were also the most dissatisfied with their jobs and suffered from high stress levels. In other words, the pain could be due to psychological or stress factors rather than simply the physical aspects of their jobs.

Rehabilitation of stroke patients

A stroke occurs when a blood clot blocks a blood vessel in the brain, causing brain cells in the area to die. If treatment is not given immediately, further cells in the surrounding areas also die. The functions that were controlled by those brain cells (such as speech, memory or movement) are then affected, depending on the area of the brain where the blood vessels were blocked. The severity of the stroke can vary from patient to patient. The effects may be very minor (and temporary), or they may lead to paralysis or death.

The main types of rehabilitation are:

- physical therapy – to improve mechanical skills such as walking, use of the hands, or balance;

- occupational therapy – to relearn the skills that are required for everyday life, such as eating, dressing and looking after oneself;
- speech therapy – to relearn how to communicate effectively.

Physiotherapy for stroke patients must begin as early as possible following the stroke in order to be effective. Improvement is slow, and recovery is difficult six months after the stroke. However, paralysed muscles must not be treated too early, or they may be damaged permanently.

Research carried out at the University of Texas and reported in *New Scientist* found that rats and monkeys that had received small brain injuries to cause paralysis of a limb suffered further injury if treatment was started immediately. The researchers surmised that glutamate, a neurotransmitter that is released during movement, was the probable cause, since, in large concentrations, it acts as a toxin. Brain damage appeared to multiply its effects. Research is now being carried out to find drugs that will block the effects of glutamate.

The expertise of the physiotherapist is vital in assessing when (and in what form) treatment should start. At the start of the treatment, the physiotherapist will prepare muscles for the more intensive treatments that will follow and will work on enabling the patient to support his or her own weight if leg muscles are affected. The later stages of physiotherapy may involve compensation for permanently damaged muscles through the introduction of aids such as walking frames. The physiotherapist may work alongside occupational therapists, speech therapists, carers and psychologists to try to prepare the patient for a return to 'normal' life.

Exercise referral schemes

Exercise referral schemes are designed to promote physical activity for people who have an existing health condition and are physically inactive. They are used to help patients suffering from a wide range of problems, including:

- coronary heart disease;
- diabetes;
- hypertension;
- mental health problems, including depression;
- musculoskeletal problems, for example, chronic lower-back pain;
- obesity;
- problems caused by falls.

Self-referral schemes

In 2016, it was reported that a new vision of primary care in England, where physiotherapists work alongside GPs as well as other health professionals, had been successfully introduced in some parts of the country. NHS Suffolk was providing physiotherapy as the first point of contact in 27 of its sites with promising results: a 30% reduction of patients suffering from musculoskeletal (MSK) issues on their GPs' caseloads. Also, a 40% reduction in patients needing knee and hip replacements has been reported.

With schemes such as these, patient needs would be met earlier, and GPs would be able to concentrate on aspects of care only they can provide. Also, allowing patients to self-refer to a physiotherapist would free up more GP appointments and also improve patient satisfaction levels.

Stand up for your health

On average, reports say that British people sit for 8.9 hours every day. Many sit for much more than that. Public Health England has issued guidance designed for employers to help them mobilise their staff to increase productivity because, in turn, this will improve the health of the workforce. They highlight certain findings that point to an increase in high blood pressure, obesity and type 2 diabetes among workers who spend most of their day sitting down.

They recommend that all workers should get between two and four hours of standing and light walking per day, that people check their movements on a regular basis and seek physiotherapy where necessary, balance sitting and standing work and, where necessary, encourage employers to equip the workplace with sit-stand desks and also employers should promote the message of a healthy work/life balance.

The role of the physio becomes especially important as the increase in activity under this scheme will mean that some people experience musculoskeletal problems. Not only will physios be responsible for the treatment of these injuries but also there is an emphasis on the profession circulating guidance on good practice and exercise techniques in order to minimise the numbers of problem cases.

This is not a new initiative and tends to be highlighted annually, certainly over the past few years. However, current research highlights the developing issue and the links with more serious illnesses, which is once again raising the profile of the need for change.

Physiotherapists given prescribing powers

There are two types of prescribing for physiotherapists:

1. **Supplementary prescribing** is the use of a written clinical management plan (CMP) to prescribe agreed medicines in partnership with a doctor. The CMP can include any licensed or unlicensed medicines and all controlled drugs.
2. **Independent prescribing** is the use of individual clinical reasoning and professional judgement to determine the nature and extent of any medicines to be used in the management of diagnosed and undiagnosed conditions. Independent prescribers may prescribe any licensed medicine from the British National Formulary, within national and local guidelines, for any condition within their area of competence within the overarching framework of human movement, performance and function.

Phil Gray, Chief Executive of the CSP, is quoted as saying, 'This is a landmark moment that will lead to patients receiving faster, more effective treatment for their condition. Physiotherapists being able to independently prescribe – for the first time anywhere in the world – will remove bureaucracy, free up time for doctors and save money for the NHS.'

Alternative therapies

Physiotherapists are becoming increasingly interested in utilising so-called 'alternative therapies' alongside traditional techniques, such as:

- acupuncture;
- Alexander technique;
- aromatherapy;
- chiropractic medicine;
- massage;
- reflex therapy.

Acupuncture

Acupuncture originated over 3,000 years ago in China. The practitioner inserts thin needles into the body at designated places in order to help alleviate or cure problems. Nowadays, this may also involve the use of small electric currents. It is thought that the needles stimulate the body's nervous system into producing its own painkilling substances. The safe delivery of acupuncture is monitored by the Acupuncture Association of Chartered Physiotherapists (AACP), a clinical interest group of the CSP.

Alexander technique

The Alexander technique is a method of releasing unwanted muscular tension throughout the body by making the patient aware of balance, posture and coordination while performing everyday actions. It is particularly associated with the performing arts.

Aromatherapy

Aromatherapy uses essential oils that are derived from plants and flowers. The oils are either vaporised and inhaled or applied directly to the body – often in conjunction with massage.

Chiropractic medicine

Chiropractic medicine aims to address the improper alignment of the vertebrae in the spine, which, it is believed, causes a number of physical disorders. Re-alignment is achieved by manipulation.

Massage

Massage is the manipulation of the soft parts of the body. Physiotherapists with a particular interest can do postgraduate training in many different types of massage. The CSP has a special interest group: Chartered Physiotherapists Interested in Massage and Soft Tissue Therapies (CPMaSTT).

Reflex therapy

Reflex therapy deals with problems within the body by targeting related points on, for example, the feet, hands or head. Reflex therapy can be arranged by consulting a chartered physiotherapist who is a member of the Association of Chartered Physiotherapists in Reflex Therapy (ACPIRT), a clinical interest group of the CSP.

8 | Massaging the results
Results day

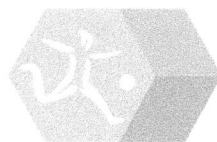

You have done all of the hard work – your personal statement, the interview, the examinations – and you are now waiting for your results, the results that will determine whether you have achieved what you need to take your university place. This chapter explains what happens when you get your results, and, if you have achieved grades that are either better or worse than expected, what other options are available to you.

When the results are available

- A levels – mid-August
- IB – early in July
- Scottish Highers – first week of August

Ask your school or college for the exact date and time that they will issue you with the results. Whichever of the exam systems you are sitting, you need to act quickly if you:

- have missed the grades or scores that you require to satisfy your firm offer;
- are not holding any offers and wish to apply through UCAS Clearing.

What to do if you have no offers: UCAS Extra

If you apply for five courses and either receive no offers or decline all the offers you get, you are eligible for UCAS Extra. Extra operates from the end of February to the beginning of July and allows you to add one additional choice at a time.

To find a course using Extra, use the UCAS search tool and the filter 'Show courses with vacancies'. Next, contact the universities and colleges listed to check if they'll consider you. It's recommended that you call the university to which you want to apply before you add the

Extra choice to check whether there is space on the course and to discuss your suitability. To apply for the new course, you need to add the details to your application.

Your chosen university will consider your application and, if this is unsuccessful, you can add another Extra choice as long as it's before July. If you have not heard back from the university within 21 days, you can add another Extra choice (again, before July).

Once you have received an offer through Extra, you'll need to either accept or decline it. Ensure that you respond by the date displayed on your homepage, or your offer will be automatically declined.

Don't worry if you don't receive the offer you'd hoped for in UCAS Extra – you can still participate in Clearing.

What to do if things go wrong during the exams

Occasionally, students will underperform in an examination through no fault of their own. This could be through distressing family circumstances (a serious illness to a family member, for example), illness in the run-up to the exam (or during the exam) or unforeseen circumstances such as late arrival to the exam due to problems with public transport. In all cases, you should inform the universities that this has happened to you immediately after the examination. You should, if possible, get your referee to give the details to the universities and provide documentary evidence, such as a letter from your GP.

What to do on results day

You can collect your results from your school or college, or you can arrange to receive them via email or post. It's a good idea to go into school or college to receive them in person so that you can get support and advice from teachers and careers advisers about your options if you need it.

UCAS receives your exam results directly and will update UCAS Hub with the outcome of your university applications on results day. The system will be busy, so you might need to be patient to find out whether you've been successful.

You'll need to have the following things ready to ensure that you can do everything you might need to on results day:

- UCAS Hub login details;
- UCAS ID number;

- UCAS Clearing number, if you go into Clearing;
- details of your offers;
- the UCAS and Clearing numbers of your chosen universities;
- a working phone and computer, so you can communicate by phone or email.

When you do get your results, one of four things will happen:

1. You receive confirmation of your place from the university you selected as your firm choice and accept it.
2. You have not met the offer from your firm choice, but you will receive confirmation from the university you selected as your insurance choice and accept it.
3. You have met and exceeded the offer made by your firm choice and decide to try to swap courses by going through Clearing (see below).
4. You have not met the requirements of any offers and need to go through Clearing.

If you have achieved the grades that meet the offer made by the university you selected as either your firm choice or insurance choice and are happy with this offer, then congratulations! You do not need to do anything. However, if you want to make use of UCAS Clearing or have not met any offers and need to use Clearing, then read on.

What to do if you exceeded the grades that you expected

If you have met and exceeded the conditional requirements of your firm choice and it has accepted you – therefore converting the conditional offer into an unconditional one – you could potentially swap your place for one on another course that you prefer. The phrase 'met and exceeded' means that if you needed BBB, you would have achieved ABB or better. It doesn't necessarily mean that you just got more UCAS points. For example, if you needed BBB and achieved A*BC, then you would have accumulated more UCAS points with A*BC than you would have if you had only achieved BBB. However, you would have still failed to meet one of your grade requirements. In cases like this, your eligibility will depend on whether your offer was based on UCAS points or grades.

If you decide to pursue a different course, you have to go through UCAS Clearing. Since more than 50,000 students get a course through Clearing, it is highly recommended that you find the course of your preference as soon as possible, as this is a first-come, first-served system.

Use the Clearing search tool to find all the available courses. Once you have found an alternative course, you will need to phone the university yourself. When you call the university, you will need to give them your UCAS personal ID number and explain straight away that you have exceeded the grades of your offers and are applying through Clearing. Be prepared to answer questions about why you really want to study that course. If they agree to accept you, and you in turn agree to accept them, this will happen during the phone call. Once you receive an offer, you can add it in your application so the college or university can officially accept you. At this stage, your status on UCAS Hub will change. Remember that if you do not find an alternative course that you want, or do not get accepted onto an alternative course, your original firm offer will still stand.

Make sure that you think carefully about the courses and universities if you decide to go through Clearing. Just because a university has higher entry requirements or is considered to be more prestigious, it does not necessarily mean that you will enjoy the course more. Consider carefully why you selected your initial firm choice and check whether your reasons are still valid and you have the same interest and passion to study a new course.

What to do if you have no confirmed offers

If you are not holding any offers, there could be several explanations.

- You may have missed the required grades of both your firm and insurance offers.
- You may have achieved the right grades but not in the right subjects.
- The university or UCAS may not have received your results. The examination boards send the results automatically to UCAS, but if you sat an exam at a different centre, for example, then this may not have happened.
- The examination system that you sat does not automatically send the results to UCAS – for instance, if you sat overseas qualifications.

In the case of achieving the right grades but not in the right subjects, contact your firm choice university to discuss this with it. Universities may revise their offer and admit you if they still have places, or if you missed the grade by only a few marks, they may ask you to try for a remark. Exam boards change the marks in only a few cases, though, and they can go down or up, so don't place all your hopes on this. If you still do not receive an offer from your firm choice university and have not received an offer from your insurance choice university, then call your insurance choice university. If, by the end of this process, you still have no offers, you will need to enter UCAS Clearing.

UCAS Clearing - Tips

Clearing is the name given to the system in which all remaining course vacancies are advertised on the UCAS website and in national newspapers. In Clearing, you contact the universities directly that have publicised course vacancies and give them your grades and UCAS ID number. If you think that you might need to use the Clearing system, it is best to be well prepared because the vacancies are filled very quickly. Clearing is typically open from July to October.

Alongside their search tool, which includes over 30,000 course options, UCAS also offers Clearing Plus, a tool that 'matches' candidates to a list of courses in UCAS Hub. If you find yourself in Clearing, it is advisable to check the 'View matches' button; if you find a course you like, select the 'I'm interested' button. If the university or college still has available places, they will contact you to discuss further and possibly make you an offer.

Advice for Clearing

- Make sure that you have your UCAS ID number and a copy of your UCAS application ready for results day.
- Remain proactive! Use the Clearing Plus tool to speed up the process of finding another place.
- You need to have access to a phone that you can use exclusively, as you may need to make a lot of calls over the course of results day.
- You also need to have access to the internet in order to access the directory of courses available through Clearing on the UCAS website. This is particularly useful as the website also has the university contact numbers that you will need to call.
- Think about the option of studying on courses that might not be identical to the one that you originally applied for but are related. For example, sociology and psychology rather than single honours psychology.

- Be ready for an impromptu telephone interview. The admissions staff may ask why you want to study on the course, and you will need to have a little bit more tact than just saying, 'because I didn't get into the course I really wanted to'. Instead, you could say something like, 'Even though I didn't get in to my firm or insurance choices I did apply/intend to apply/visit during the open day/know that the course has a good student satisfaction rating in the Guardian, etc.'

If you decide to retake your A levels

If you have not achieved the grades that you needed for your chosen universities and do not want to take the available Clearing places, you could consider retaking one or more A levels. In the days when most examination boards offered January sittings, retaking might have meant studying for one term to boost the grade. The period from January to September could then be used to earn money, gain more work experience or travel the world. But, apart from international A levels, A level exams are now only available in June, and so retaking will involve studying for another year, so you need to be sure that your university aspirations are genuine enough to give you the motivation to add this extra year to your studies. As the A level system is now fully reformed, barring the last Phase Three legacy-subject examinations, you will need to retake the entire two-year qualification again and therefore plan to be able to do this in just a single year – you do not want a repeat of the examination if you are underprepared.

Speak to your teachers about the implications of retaking your exams. Some independent sixth-form colleges provide specialist advice and teaching for students. Interviews to discuss this are free and carry no obligation to enrol in a course, so it is worth taking the time to talk to their staff before you embark on A level retakes. Many further education colleges also offer retake courses, and some schools will allow students to return to resit subjects, either as external examination candidates or by repeating a year.

If you decide to reapply

Universities are usually happy to consider students who are reapplying, either because they did not get the required grades the first time around or because they did not receive any offers of places. It is worth contacting the university to check whether this is the case. Some will have policies on grade requirements for retake candidates, while others might ask for evidence of any extenuating circumstances that may have affected the previous application.

TIP!

- If there were extenuating circumstances that affected your application, include a brief mention of this in the personal statement ('I was disappointed not to have achieved the required grades, because my studies were affected by illness, but this has made me even more determined to become an engineer') but leave the details to the referee.
- If you are retaking, you can use the extra term or extra year to add weight to your application, for example, by gaining more work experience, taking up a new subject, enrolling in evening classes that are relevant to your application and furthering your reading.

9 | The fifth metatarsal
Non-standard applications

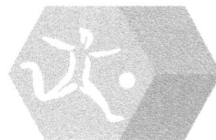

So far, this book has been concerned with the 'standard' applicant: the UK resident who is studying at least two science subjects at A level or Scottish Highers, International Baccalaureate, Irish Leaving Certificate and BTEC courses and who is applying from school or who is retaking immediately after disappointing results. This chapter outlines the application process for 'non-standard' applicants.

The main non-standard categories are as follows.

Students who have not studied science A levels

If you decide that you would like to study physiotherapy after having already started on a combination of A levels that does not fit the subject requirements for entry to university, you have three choices.

1. You can spend an extra year studying science A levels at a sixth-form college that offers one-year A level courses. You should discuss your particular circumstances with prospective colleges in order to select suitable courses. You need to be aware that only very able students can cover A level Chemistry and Biology in a single year with good results.
2. You can follow a Foundation course at a university that will then allow you to study a related degree course afterwards. For details of Foundation courses, you should contact universities.
3. You can enrol in an Access course that is recognised by the universities you wish to apply to. Each university will have different policies about Access courses – you should contact the physiotherapy departments directly.

International students

The competition for the few places available to international students is fierce, and you would be wise to discuss your application informally with the university before submitting it. In general, overseas applicants will find it difficult to gain a place unless they can offer qualifications that are recognised by the universities, such as A levels or the IB. There are, however, bridging qualifications purposely designed for international students that can qualify students for entry into Physiotherapy courses, such as the NCUK International Foundation Year in Science.

Information about qualifications can be obtained from British Council offices, British embassies and the universities that offer physiotherapy courses. Overseas students are liable for the full cost of tuition. For physiotherapy, the fees vary greatly depending on the university. They can range from £14,950 to £35,800 per year. The UCAS website has a section for international students that describes in detail the application process and deadlines.

English language qualifications

In order to begin a university degree in this country, you are required to have an accredited English language qualification if you are an international student. This is because it is essential that you are able to understand the course and what is being taught to you throughout your studies.

You should aim to achieve at least IELTS (International English Language Testing System) 6.5 to 7.0 in order to begin a university course and certainly no less than 6.5 in each band. Most universities will set the boundary higher, commonly at 7.0 now, in order to discourage some applications. If you would like further information on IELTS, please visit www.ielts.org.

While IELTS is the most commonly requested English language certificate by universities in the UK, there are a wide range of other English language tests now available, and since the pandemic, UK universities have become more flexible on the certificates they will accept. Other examples of language certificates that will be considered include PTE Academic, TOEFL, LanguageCert, Skills for English and Duolingo. Nevertheless, it remains important to check with your chosen universities that they will accept a certain English language certificate before booking and paying for the test.

Visa requirements

If you require a visa to be in the UK and your course is longer than six months, which Physiotherapy courses invariably are, then you will need to apply for a student visa. In order to do this, the university you are accepted by will request from you various pieces of information, including your education transcripts and passport. They will produce a Confirmation of Acceptance of Studies (CAS) letter for you once you have given them all the information and paid a specific deposit; you will take the CAS letter to the UK embassy in your country in order to obtain a visa for studying. Do not delay in this process, as obtaining a visa can take time, which varies from country to country.

Mature students

Physiotherapy courses are popular with older students, and the universities tend to have a flexible and encouraging approach to students over the age of 21.

Nowadays, more than half of the physiotherapy student cohort is mature students. Work experience is key, as it points to you being a strong candidate and having researched the course properly.

Graduates

A 2.i degree (or higher) along with at least a grade B in A level Biology is normally required for graduates applying for physiotherapy. Most universities ask graduates to take a year out between the final year of their first degree course and the start of the Physiotherapy course in order to get work experience. This allows them to demonstrate that they are serious about a career in physiotherapy.

Applicants with no suitable academic qualifications

Candidates are likely to be asked to sit for at least two A levels, one of which will be Biology, and to achieve B grades or higher. There are also some Access courses that can lead to an offer of a place to study physiotherapy; applicants should liaise with universities to confirm suitability.

The main difficulty facing those coming late to the idea of studying physiotherapy is that they rarely have a scientific background. They face the daunting task of studying science A levels and need very careful counselling before they embark on what will, inevitably, be quite a tough programme. Independent sixth-form colleges provide this counselling as part of their normal interview procedure.

Access courses

A proportion of colleges of further education offer Access courses suitable for physiotherapy. One well-known example is the course at the College of West Anglia in King's Lynn. Primarily (but not exclusively) aimed at health professionals, they offer a full-time, one-year course in Access to Science and Nursing. It should be noted there are also other providers.

The course that you take might be Access to Science, to Health Studies, to Physiotherapy or to Medical Sciences, but you must cover cardiovascular, pulmonary and skeletal muscle physiology at level 3. Some universities will ask for biology or human biology. You should contact the specific university to find out exactly which Access course it recognises.

You should contact the university admissions tutors or look on the university websites for advice. There is a strong case for suggesting that those people getting into universities are the ones who put in the work beforehand by talking to the universities. If you have a question, ask it – you will get an answer that you can then base your decision on.

Physiotherapy Degree Apprenticeships

A Degree-standard Apprenticeship in physiotherapy is a new entry route into the profession. To be considered for a Degree Apprenticeship, you will first need to apply for an apprentice position with a healthcare provider; vacancies can be found on the NHS Jobs website and Find an Apprenticeship website. The scheme is primarily a work-based programme, developing the skills and behaviour a student will need to become a physiotherapist. An end-point assessment (EPA) will need to be passed in order to complete the course.

Once you've successfully completed a programme approved by the HCPC, you will then be eligible to apply for registration with the HCPC. Once registered as a practitioner, you'll be required to retain your name on the register by keeping your knowledge and skills up to date through engaging in CPD and paying an annual retention fee.

Students with disabilities and special educational needs

Universities welcome applications from students who have physical or other disabilities or special educational needs, and they have well-established support systems in place to provide assistance and special facilities. The services offered can help with a wide range of disabilities, including sensory (visual/hearing) impairment, mental health difficulties, mobility impairment, dexterity impairment, Asperger's syndrome, or other autistic spectrum disorders or chronic medical conditions (e.g. dyslexia or dyspraxia). In all cases, you should contact the universities directly before you apply to explain your particular needs and requirements. They will be able to give you information on how they can help you. The website www.disabilityrightsuk.org contains useful links and information.

10 | Make no bones about it
Fees and funding

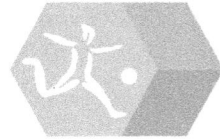

Whether undertaking an undergraduate or postgraduate course, the cost of studying is considerable. This has been exacerbated in recent years by rises in living costs due to inflation alongside the cost of university tuition fees. According to the UK Parliament's House of Commons Library, on average, students commencing their studies in 2022 were likely to accrue a student loan debt of £45,600.

When considering levels of student debt, it is easy to become disheartened and think that university study is not for you. What all students must remember is that tuition fees do not have to be paid up front; in fact, most students receive student loans to cover this cost. In addition, the loans do not start to be paid back until you are earning over a certain amount. However, it can be a real challenge for many students to pay for living costs, such as rent and food, so it is vital to be aware of how you will meet these expenses.

Undertaking any university course should only be done after seriously considering the overall cost and carefully examining your ability to be fully committed to your study.

Fees

UK students

As each UK nation sets its own fees, the tuition fee that students have to pay for undergraduate courses will depend on where you live and where you intend to study. From 1 August 2025, the maximum annual tuition fee that providers will be allowed to charge will be £9,535, as part of the government's Teaching Excellence Framework (TEF), which assesses universities and colleges on the quality of their teaching.

There are a number of variations between the systems in England, Scotland, Wales and Northern Ireland, which can result in significant differences between the fees that are ultimately paid by students. In the autumn of 2024, the UK government announced that the tuition fee cap in England would be increasing from £9,250 to £9,535 for the 2025–26 academic year; this was followed by announcements by the

Welsh and Scottish governments that they would bring their fees in line with England. Northern Ireland is set to increase tuition fees from £4,750 to £4,855 for 2025 entry. Therefore, the current rules are as follows, although they may be subject to change in the future.

- Students in England and Wales are required to pay a maximum of £9,535 if they are studying in England, Scotland, Wales or Northern Ireland.
- Students from Scotland who study at Scottish universities are not required to pay tuition fees (or, rather, tuition fees of £1,820 for 2025 entry are covered by the Student Awards Agency for Scotland [SAAS] for students who qualify for home student status). Scottish students have to pay fees of up to £9,535 if they study in England, Wales or Northern Ireland.
- Students living in Northern Ireland pay up to £4,855 if they attend university in Northern Ireland, up to £9,535 if they study in England, Scotland or Wales.

EU and non-EU international students

At present, EU students are charged the same fees as those charged to non-EU international students, which are significantly higher than those charged to UK students and are determined by each university.

Some students from the EU may be eligible for some support in terms of student loans from the UK government, but this is dependent on a number of factors, so it is best to check personal eligibility. Students from the Republic of Ireland are exempt from paying higher fees and are eligible for home fee status.

Living expenses

Your living expenses include the cost of your accommodation, food, clothes, travel and equipment, leisure and social activities – plus possible extras like field trips and study visits, if these aren't covered by the tuition fees.

Check university and college websites for information about possible living costs. Some are more informative than others and give breakdowns under various headings such as accommodation, food and daily travel. Others go even further and give typical weekly, monthly or annual spends.

If you're living away from home, accommodation will make up the largest proportion of your living costs. There is likely to be a range of accommodation options – from a standard room in university halls through to privately rented accommodation – with a range of price points. You'll probably be surprised when you do some research to find that the cheapest and most expensive towns are not as you might have expected; the cost of accommodation often depends on how much of it is available in a particular area.

When choosing accommodation, it is essential to consider its location and factor in the cost of travel to your university or college. It is also important to find out what's included in the accommodation costs (such as utilities, personal property insurance and Wi-Fi) and whether it is possible to pay for accommodation during term time only.

Funding your studies

How do you fund your time in higher education? Don't ignore this question and leave it until the last minute! You will need to think carefully about how to budget for several years' costs – and you need to know what help you might get from:

- the government;
- your family or partner;
- paid part-time work;
- other sources, such as bursaries and scholarships.

This chapter gives a brief overview of a complicated funding situation, which can vary according to where you come from and where you plan to study. For more details about the different types of funding available and how to apply for them, check your regional student finance website:

- www.gov.uk/contact-student-finance-england
- www.saas.gov.uk
- www.studentfinanceni.co.uk
- www.studentfinancewales.co.uk

Tuition fee loans

For UK students, tuition fees can be covered by taking out a tuition fee loan, which will be paid directly to your university or college at the start of each year of your course. You are effectively given a loan by the government that you repay through your income tax from the April after you finish your course but only once your earnings reach a certain threshold. Currently, these income thresholds stand at:

- £25,000 per year for students from England;
- £27,295 per year for students from Wales;
- £31,395 for students from Scotland (who go to university outside of Scotland);
- £24,990 per year for students from Northern Ireland.

So, if you never reach this threshold, you will not have to repay the fees. In addition, any outstanding balance on your loan will be cancelled after a certain period of time if you have not already cleared it in full. The length of time depends on the rules at the time you took out the loan. For students in England who started their studies after August 2023, the repayment period was extended to 40 years (from 30 years), so it is recommended that students in other regions keep a close eye on any developments with respect to the length of the loan repayment period. At the time of writing, the loan repayment term is 30 years for students from Wales and Scotland and 25 years for students from Northern Ireland.

The current situation regarding repayments is that you repay 9% of anything you earn over the annual income threshold.

The interest rate charged on student loans depends on what repayment plan you are on, but for students in England on Plan 5, it is currently set at 4.3%.

Maintenance loans

In addition to a tuition fee loan, all students can apply for a maintenance or living cost loan. All students are entitled to a maintenance loan, which is repayable in the same way. The amount you can borrow will be dependent on your household income – in other words, it is means-tested. 'Household income' refers to your family's gross annual income (their income before tax). With the exception of loans available to Scottish students, the amount you can claim also varies depending on your living situation, with the maximum loan being available to students living away from home in London.

Each regional student finance website includes a finance calculator tool that will give an estimate of the finance you would be eligible for based on your family income and other factors, and it is well worth looking at this before planning your budget.

England (2025-26)
The maximum annual maintenance loan in England:

- £8,877 for those living in the family home;
- £10,544 for those living away from home (£13,762 in London).

Wales (2025-26)
In Wales, students can get a combination of a maintenance grant, which they do not have to pay back, and a repayable maintenance loan. Both are means-tested, but all students will get a grant of at least £1,000.

The combined total amounts available from maintenance loans and grants in Wales are:

- £10,480 for those living in the family home;
- £12,345 for those living away from home (£15,415 in London).

Scotland (2024-25)

In Scotland, all students can get a repayable maintenance loan, and those eligible will receive a non-repayable bursary (grant) to cover living expenses. These are as follows (all figures per year):

- Household income up to £20,999: £2,000 bursary and £7,000 loan;
- Household income £21,000–£23,999: £1,125 bursary and £7,000 loan;
- Household income £24,000: £33,999: £500 bursary and £7,000 loan;
- Household income £34,000 and above: no bursary and £6,000 loan.

Unlike the rest of the UK, household income for Scottish students is measured on the income bands listed above rather than exact household income.

From the 2024–25 academic year, an additional new 'special support' loan of £2,400 is available to all full-time students. Unlike the maintenance loan and bursary, this is not means-tested, but it is repayable.

Northern Ireland (2025-26)

The maximum annual maintenance loan in Northern Ireland:

- £6,300 for those living in the family home;
- £8,132 for those living away from home (£11,391 in London).

In addition, you may be eligible for a non-repayable maintenance grant if your household income is below £41,065. This is paid alongside any maintenance loan you qualify for and is up to £3,475.

Additional funding

NHS bursaries

Home students in England might be eligible to apply for an NHS Learning Support Fund (LSF) of £5,000 per academic year. The NHS LSF offers financial assistance to eligible students in four key areas, depending on individual circumstances. Students can receive a training grant of £5,000 annually or a pro rata amount for part-time study, with an additional special subject payment of £1,000 for certain courses. Those with dependent children under 15 or 17, if they have special educational needs, can access parental support, providing £2,000 per year or a pro rata amount for part-time students. Travel and dual accommodation expenses allow reimbursement for extra costs incurred during placements. If facing unexpected financial challenges, students may apply for up to £3,000 through the exceptional support fund.

In Wales, students may receive a non-means-tested NHS grant, currently around £1,000 per year, and are eligible for a means-tested NHS bursary to help with day-to-day living costs. All new and prospective students are eligible to apply, and students who are awarded these bursaries can also apply for student loans.

If you've been living in Northern Ireland for the last three years, you can apply for an income-assessed bursary to assist with living costs for health professional degrees there.

To address national workforce needs, the Scottish Government tasked NHS Education for Scotland with implementing the Funded Places Scheme. This initiative supports students committed to pursuing a career within NHS Scotland by enabling them to enrol in an MSc (pre-registration) Physiotherapy programme at a Scottish university.

Sponsorship

Sponsorship is also sometimes available from prospective future employers; the armed forces are particularly well known to support students through their training. If you wish to apply for sponsorship from a specific sports club or national body – and bear in mind that some of them will not advertise such schemes – then it is often best to get in touch personally in writing, stating your aims and career aspirations and the course onto which you have been accepted to study.

11 | Exercise the mind
Useful information and further resources

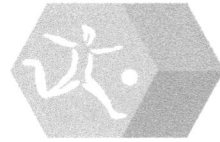

You are advised to check the UCAS Handbook or website for information on courses and universities before applying.

Universities offering physiotherapy degrees

University of Bedfordshire
Tel: 01234 400400
Website: www.beds.ac.uk

University College Birmingham
Tel: 0121 604 1000
Website: www.ucb.ac.uk

University of Birmingham
Tel: 0121 414 3344
Website: www.birmingham.ac.uk

Bournemouth University
Tel: 01202 524111
Website: www.bournemouth.ac.uk

University of Bradford
Tel: 01274 232323
Website: www.bradford.ac.uk

University of Brighton
Tel: 01273 600900
Website: www.brighton.ac.uk

Bristol, University of the West of England
Tel: 0117 965 6261
Website: www.uwe.ac.uk

Brunel University
Tel: 01895 274000
Website: www.brunel.ac.uk

Canterbury Christ Church University
Tel: 01227 928000
Website: www.canterbury.ac.uk

Cardiff University
Tel: 029 2087 4000
Website: www.cardiff.ac.uk

University of Central Lancashire
Tel: 01772 201201
Website: www.uclan.ac.uk

University of Chichester
Tel: 01243 816000
Website: www.chi.ac.uk

City St George's, University of London
Tel: 020 7040 5060
Website: www.citystgeorges.ac.uk

Coventry University
Tel: 024 7765 7688
Website: www.coventry.ac.uk

University of Cumbria
Tel: 01228 616234 (Carlisle)
Website: www.cumbria.ac.uk

University of East Anglia
Tel: 01603 456161
Website: www.uea.ac.uk

University of East London
Tel: 020 8223 3000
Website: www.uel.ac.uk

University of Essex
Tel: 01206 873333
Website: www.essex.ac.uk

Glasgow Caledonian University
Tel: 0141 331 3000
Website: www.gcu.ac.uk

University of Gloucestershire
Tel: 01242 714700
Website: www.glos.ac.uk

University of Greater Manchester
Tel: 01204 900600
Website: www.bolton.ac.uk

University of Hertfordshire
Tel: 01707 284000
Website: www.herts.ac.uk

University of Huddersfield
Tel: 01484 422288
Website: www.hud.ac.uk

University of Hull
Tel: 01482 346311
Website: www.hull.ac.uk

Keele University
Tel: 01782 734010
Website: www.keele.ac.uk

King's College London
Tel: 020 7836 5454
Website: www.kcl.ac.uk

Leeds Beckett University
Tel: 0113 812 0000
Website: www.leedsbeckett.ac.uk

University of Leicester
Tel: 0116 252 2522
Website: www.le.ac.uk

University of Liverpool
Tel: 0151 794 5927
Website: www.liv.ac.uk

London South Bank University
Tel: 020 7815 7815
Website: www.lsbu.ac.uk

Manchester Metropolitan University
Tel: 0161 247 6969
Website: www.mmu.ac.uk

Newman University Birmingham
Tel: 0121 476 1181
Website: www.newman.ac.uk

Northumbria University
Tel: 0191 406 0901
Website: www.northumbria.ac.uk

University of Nottingham
Tel: 0115 951 5151
Website: www.nottingham.ac.uk

Oxford Brookes University
Tel: 01865 741111
Website: www.brookes.ac.uk

Plymouth University
Tel: 01752 600600
Website: www.plymouth.ac.uk

Plymouth Marjon University
Tel: 01752 636700
Website: www.marjon.ac.uk

Queen Margaret University, Edinburgh
Tel: 0131 474 0000
Website: www.qmu.ac.uk

Robert Gordon University, Aberdeen
Tel: 01224 262000
Website: www.rgu.ac.uk

University of Salford
Tel: 0161 295 0000
Website: www.salford.ac.uk

Sheffield Hallam University
Tel: 0114 225 5555
Website: www.shu.ac.uk

South Bank University, London
Tel: 020 7815 7815
Website: www.lsbu.ac.uk

University of Southampton
Tel: 023 8059 5000
Website: www.southampton.ac.uk

University of South Wales
Tel: 03455 767778
Website: www.southwales.ac.uk

St Mary's Twickenham
Tel: 020 8240 4000
Website: www.stmarys.ac.uk

University of Suffolk
Tel: 01473 338833
Website: www.uos.ac.uk

University of Sunderland
Tel: 0191 515 3000
Website: www.sunderland.ac.uk

Teesside University
Tel: 01642 218121
Website: www.tees.ac.uk

University of Ulster
Tel: 028 7012 3456
Website: www.ulster.ac.uk

University of Winchester
Tel: 01962 841515
Website: www.winchester.ac.uk

University of Wolverhampton
Tel: 01902 321000
Website: www.wlv.ac.uk

University of Worcester
Tel: 01905 855000
Website: www.worcester.ac.uk

Wrexham University
Tel: 01978 290666
Website: www.wrexham.ac.uk

York St John University
Tel: 01904 624624
Website: www.yorksj.ac.uk

Useful resources

Chartered Society of Physiotherapy

An essential starting point is the CSP's website (www.csp.org.uk). It carries detailed information about careers in physiotherapy and recognised courses. The CSP also produces many useful booklets about physiotherapy. It can be contacted at:

Chartered Society of Physiotherapy
14 Bedford Row
London WC1R 4ED
Tel: 020 7306 6666

The CSP publishes a magazine, *Frontline*, aimed at practising physiotherapists. The magazine contains articles of interest and is a useful way of keeping up to date with current issues and new developments. There is also a large jobs section – a good way to make contact with physiotherapy practices if you are looking for work experience.

Other societies

Irish Society of Chartered Physiotherapists
13 Adelaide Road
Dublin
D02 P950
Ireland
Tel: +353 1 5240 931
Website: www.iscp.ie

Royal College of Occupational Therapists
106–14 Borough High Street
London SE1 1LB
Tel: 020 3141 4600
Website: www.rcot.co.uk

Royal College of Podiatry
2nd Floor, Quartz House
207 Providence Square
Mill Street
London SE1 2EW
Tel: 020 7234 8620
Website: www.rcpod.org.uk

World Federation of Occupational Therapists
Website: www.wfot.org

UCAS

For information on university applications, contact UCAS (www.ucas
.com). The UCAS website has a search facility that will enable you to
check the latest entrance requirements for all universities that offer
Physiotherapy courses. Application materials can be obtained from:

UCAS
Rosehill
New Barn Lane
Cheltenham GL52 3LZ

Other useful addresses

Department for Economy (Northern Ireland)
Netherleigh
Massey Avenue
Belfast BT4 2JP
Tel: 028 9052 9900
Website: www.economy-ni.gov.uk

NHS (England) Student Bursaries
Tel: 0300 330 1345
Website: www.nhsbsa.nhs.uk/nhs-bursary-students

Student Awards Agency Scotland
Saughton House
Broomhouse Drive
Edinburgh EH11 3UT
Website: www.saas.gov.uk

Student Awards Services (NHS Wales)
Floor 4
Companies House
Crown Way
Cardiff CF14 3UB
Tel: 029 2090 3700
Website: www.nwsspstudentfinance.wales.nhs.uk/home

Useful websites

Examination boards

www.aqa.org.uk
www.ets.org/toefl
www.ielts.org
www.ocr.org.uk
http://qualifications.pearson.com
www.wjec.co.uk

Online physiotherapy information

www.evidence.nhs.uk
www.lifemark.ca
www.naidex.co.uk
www.thephysiotherapysite.co.uk

University league tables

www.theguardian.com/education/universityguide

Work experience

www.prospects.ac.uk

Fees and funding

www.studentfinanceni.co.uk
www.studentfinancewales.co.uk

www.ucas.com/undergraduate/student-life/getting-student-support/
undergraduate-student-support
www.gov.uk/education/funding-and-finance-for-students

Further reading

Books on careers/university applications

How to Complete Your UCAS Application, Ryan Moran and UCAS, MPW Guides/Trotman Education.

University Degree Course Offers: The essential guide to winning your place at university, Brian Heap, Trotman Education

Books on physiotherapy

There are numerous textbooks covering all aspects of physiotherapy. Most of these are aimed at undergraduates or physiotherapy professionals. The following will give A level (or the equivalent) students an overview of what studying physiotherapy would entail:

A Practical Guide to Sports Injuries, Malcolm T.F. Read, Butterworth-Heinemann

Principles and Practice of Physical Therapy, William E. Arnould-Taylor, Stanley Thornes

12| Don't be bone idle

Glossary

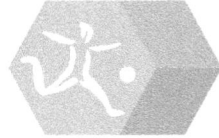

CCG
Clinical commissioning group.

CfWI
The Centre for Workforce Intelligence.

CPD
Continuing professional development.

CSP
The Chartered Society of Physiotherapy.

CTD
Cumulative trauma disorder.

ESWT
Extracorporeal shockwave therapy.

Frontline
CSP magazine.

Gait re-education
Learning to walk with a normal pattern again.

HCPC
Health and Care Professions Council.

HESA
Higher Education Statistics Agency.

HPAT
Health Professions Admission Test (Ireland).

Hydrotherapy
Using water in treating pain relief and illness.

Infrared and ultraviolet radiation
Used to warm damaged muscles and speed up healing.

IPE
Inter-professional education.

MCSP
Member of the Chartered Society of Physiotherapy.

MDT
Multidisciplinary team.

NHS
National Health Service.

OOS
Occupational overuse syndrome.

PBL
Problem-based learning.

PBPL
Practice-based professional learning.

Personal statement
Part of the UCAS application (4,000 characters with spaces), aimed at persuading universities to accept your application.

RSI
Repetitive strain injury.

SRP
State-Registered Physiotherapist.

Tennis elbow
Calcification of a tendon

UCAS
The Universities and Colleges Admissions Service.

Ultrasound
Using sound waves to break down scar tissue and reduce inflammation.

WRMSD
Work-related musculoskeletal disorder.

WRULD
Work-related upper limb disorder.

Postscript

If you have any comments or questions arising out of this book, we and the staff of MPW would be very happy to answer them. You can contact us at the addresses below.

Good luck with your applications!
Aaron Ghuman

MPW (London)
90–92 Queen's Gate
London SW7 5AB
Tel: 020 7835 1355
Email: london@mpw.ac.uk

MPW (Cambridge)
3–4 Brookside
Cambridge CB2 1JE
Tel: 01223 350158
Email: cambridge@mpw.ac.uk

MPW (Birmingham)
16–18 Greenfield Crescent
Edgbaston
Birmingham B15 3AU
Tel: 0121 454 9637
Email: birmingham@mpw.ac.uk

www.ingramcontent.com/pod-product-compliance
Lightning Source LLC
Chambersburg PA
CBHW040136270326
41927CB00019B/3409